PSYCHOLOGY FOR NURSES AND THE CARING PROFESSIONS

SOCIAL SCIENCE FOR NURSES AND THE CARING PROFESSIONS

Series Editor: Professor Pamela Abbott
University of Derby, Mickleover, Derby, UK

Current and forthcoming titles

Psychology for Nurses and the Caring Professions
Sheila Payne and Jan Walker

Sociology for Nurses and the Caring Professions
Joan Chandler

Social Policy for Nurses and the Caring Professions
Louise Ackers and Pamela Abbott

PSYCHOLOGY FOR NURSES AND THE CARING PROFESSIONS

Sheila Payne and
Jan Walker

OPEN UNIVERSITY PRESS
Buckingham • Philadelphia

Open University Press
Celtic Court
22 Ballmoor
Buckingham
MK18 1XW

and
1900 Frost Road, Suite 101
Bristol, PA 19007, USA

First Published 1996
Reprinted 1997

A catalogue record of this book is available from the British Library

ISBN 0 335 19410 9 (pb)   0 335 19411 7 (hb)

Library of Congress Cataloging-in-Publication Data
Payne, Sheila, 1954–
    Psychology for nurses and the caring professions / Sheila Payne
and Jan Walker.
        p. cm. — (Social science for nurses and the caring
professions)
    Includes bibliographical references and index.
    ISBN 0–335–19411–7 (hb)   ISBN 0–335–19410–9 (pb)
    1. Clinical health psychology. 2. Patients—Psychology.
3. Nursing—Psychological aspects. I. Walker, Jan, 1946–
II. Title. III. Series.
R726.7.P38 1995
610'.19—dc20   95–14761
                                                                CIP

Typeset by Graphicraft Typesetters Limited, Hong Kong
Printed in Great Britain by Redwood Books, Trowbridge

CONTENTS

SERIES EDITOR'S PREFACE

It is now widely recognized that the Social Sciences are central to Nurse Education. Nursing as a profession needs to ground itself in an understanding of social structures and relations, state policies and their constraints on the behaviour and experience of individuals and groups. The series of which this is one volume aims to provide nurses and others in the caring professions with lively and accessible introductions to the issues and debates within the social science disciplines.

Psychology for Nurses and the Caring Professions is a relevant and readable introduction to psychology, aimed in the first instance at nurses but relevant to a much wider professional audience. It not only enables the reader to gain an understanding of the relevance of psychology to nursing but more generally introduces many of the central debates and ideas of psychology, using examples which will be of interest to nurses and others. In other words, it introduces psychology as a discipline whose issues and theories and whose insights are of relevance in their own right.

Recognizing that the relevance of psychology to nursing is not necessarily immediately apparent, the authors explicitly set out to demonstrate the value of a psychological understanding for health care workers. Their aim is not to provide nurses with a set of techniques that can be followed in order to improve practice – though psychology *is* relevant to caring practice, as this book shows – but to introduce them to a way of thinking about and understanding individuals and social relationships. The insights that are gained will provide techniques that can be used in daily practice, but, more importantly, they will enable nurses and others in the caring professions to make more sense of the lives of the individuals with whom they are working and extend the range of ways in which they can help them. Specifically, psychology will help to inform them about vulnerable groups with whom they work – babies, children, older people, people with learning disabilities and those having trouble coping with the strains and demands of contemporary life. It will also provide insight into the problems and difficulties of coping with long-term chronic illness and the complex ways in which attitudes and habits are formed and become resistant to change.

The authors are both chartered psychologists and both qualified nurses. They have considerable experience of teaching psychology, to nursing students among others. They are able to use this experience to write an accessible and relevant introduction to psychology for nurses on both pre- and post-registration courses, and for members of other caring professions.

Pamela Abbott

PREFACE

This book aims to encourage health professionals to use psychological knowledge in their clinical practice. The authors are both nurses and health psychologists, and we have drawn heavily on both our clinical experience as nurses and our research interests as psychologists.

Knowledgeable readers will identify from looking at the contents of the book that whole areas of psychology, such as information processing and individual differences, have been omitted. While we acknowledge that these have a number of important implications for, and applications in, health care – for example, in the introduction of new technology and the use of psychometric testing – we have taken the deliberate decision to omit these issues in favour of those which relate more directly to inter-personal care. We would direct interested readers to other general and specific texts on these subjects. Other areas of psychology have been dealt with in a relatively cursory manner, while those which are covered in detail include health, social and developmental psychology.

The topics are chosen to illustrate some of the problems which are currently faced within psychology itself and we have tried to highlight contentious issues throughout. Needless to say, the coverage also reflects our biases and interests. In many situations, there are no clear-cut solutions and readers are invited, through exercises, to draw their own conclusions.

We have tried to make this book user-friendly by incorporating current research in focused discussions, exercises and detailing linkages with references to material in other parts of the book. Supplementary reading is recommended throughout. It is hoped that lecturers will add their own sources to the lists provided to present their own perspectives on the issues and raise different issues for consideration.

A glossary of terms is provided at the end of the book. This covers definitions of all the terms highlighted in bold throughout the text. References to recent research are given in the standard format, so that students will be encouraged to look up the originals and learn to use a correct academic style. However, references to pre-war and classic experiments, which are commonly reported in standard introductory texts, are omitted on the assumption that students are more likely to refer to secondary sources for these.

We hope that this book will not only function as a text to support psychology courses in health care, but will foster an interest in readers in the way psychological processes influence making sense of health and illness.

Sheila Payne
Jan Walker

INTRODUCTION TO PSYCHOLOGY

What is psychology?

Psychology is the study of behaviour and mental processes. The relative balance in focus between behaviour and mind has varied over time as psychology has developed during the last century and the definition of psychology has tended to reflect the theories and concerns of the period. Psychology is a huge subject, but in this book we will be selecting those aspects which are of most direct relevance to nurses, midwives and therapists. Recently, a separate branch of psychology called **health psychology** has come into being and we will draw examples from this discipline to illustrate the applications of psychology and psychological theory within health care practice.

Every day in conversation, on television and in newspapers people use the word psychology or make psychological statements. In hospitals and clinics, nurses and health care professionals make psychological judgements about their patients and colleagues and attribute meanings to their actions. For example, an individual may be described as having a 'huge ego' when they continually boast about their achievements in order to elicit praise. However, this is 'pop' psychology and not the type of psychology which you will be introduced to in this book.

Psychology is an academic discipline which uses theories (logical explanations) to make predictions or understand how people behave and think. Psychologists design and undertake carefully planned research studies to test out their ideas. Traditionally, they have used animals as well as humans as subjects for their research, although animals are rarely used nowadays. Psychologists use experiments, observations and other scientific methods to collect information about people. Only after a careful analysis of this information (data), will they make statements about how processes such as memory occur. Even then, they will continue to collect new information which may mean they have to modify their theories over time. Psychologists are interested in processes which occur over very variable time-spans – from a few milliseconds, as in a visual reaction time experiment, to an entire lifespan, as in developmental theory.

Psychology in health care

Psychology can contribute to our understanding of ourselves and our relationships with other people if it is applied in an informed way. Nurses, midwives and therapists spend most, if not all, of their working lives with other people. These include: persons seeking health advice or care or who have a health problem (the clients or patients); carers, such as other family members; colleagues within multidisciplinary teams who have different professional backgrounds; students; ancillary health workers, and many more. To work successfully in a health care context involves understanding not only how individuals function but how they interact with each other.

There are three main reasons why psychology is relevant to health care. First, it informs us about the needs of potentially vulnerable groups in society. These include babies and children, elderly people, those who have learning difficulties, those who experience social and economic disadvantage, those who cannot cope with contemporary life, and the list goes on. In fact, we all belong to one or more of these groups at some time in our lives. Second, at the end of the twentieth century, chronic illnesses such as cardiovascular diseases, cancer, respiratory diseases, degenerative conditions (including arthritis and dementia) are major concerns. Thus people are likely to experience illnesses that require long-term care and treatment which may have profound consequences for their ability to function and for their quality of life. Finally, it has been suggested that the lifestyles people lead have important implications for the development of subsequent illness. In 1992, the British Government produced a document entitled *The Health of the Nation,* which emphasized 'the need for people to change their behaviour – whether on smoking, alcohol consumption, exercise, diet, avoidance of accidents and, with AIDS, sexual behaviour' (DoH 1992a: iv). Lifestyle implies an individual pattern of behaviours. Behaviour change has long been a key focus within psychology, and understanding lifestyle and health-related behaviour change is a central theme within health psychology.

Studying psychology

Psychology is a core subject for the health care professions, along with sociology and physiology, but it can be difficult to follow if its relevance is not easily understood. Psychology has various and somewhat contradictory reputations. On one hand, it is seen by some as a difficult subject to comprehend; on the other, it is viewed by many as common sense. Part of this difficulty lies in the fact that there are very basic philosophical differences in how people understand the world and the nature of reality. Without going into too much depth, 'hard' scientists, including those who work within biomedical science, believe that there is an absolute reality which we can learn about through experiments and other means, and thus establish the 'facts'. Others, including many philosophers and sociologists, believe that our experience of the world is socially constructed. This means that there are no 'facts' as such but that people share meanings which may change over time and vary in different settings. Psychology lies somewhere in between these viewpoints and includes models which, as you will see, reflect either position.

Exercise

How many explanations have been offered to explain mental 'illness' over the centuries? Why was it referred to as an Illness? How many of these explanations appear to be 'scientific' and how many can be described as 'social constructions' based upon the prevailing understanding of their time? (You will find a further discussion of some of these issues in Chapter 2.)

It is important to understand how human beings function when they are healthy so that we can help them when they become ill or disabled. Functioning as a person involves social and psychological aspects, as well as having fully functioning body systems. It was Descartes, in the seventeenth century, who suggested that the mind and the body could be understood as independent parts. In Western science, this has given rise to discrete disciplines, such as physiology, psychology and sociology, which study different aspects of people in quite separate ways. Most health studies courses are now trying to put these parts back together so that students learn about and treat people in an integrated or holistic way.

Because psychology is a relatively young science, there is a range of diverse and sometimes contradictory theories and research evidence. This means that there are few accepted facts and little received wisdom, and that there are many different explanations of how human beings function. Psychologists like to debate with each other the merits of different ideas and approaches. When you study psychology, you become part of this debate. So think carefully about what you read, ask lots of questions (of yourself or others) and challenge the basic assumptions.

Application of psychological theories

The following section will introduce you to the main theoretical approaches in psychology. In order to give you an understanding of how they can be used and applied in health care, they will be related to the issues raised in a brief case study of Ann, outlined below.

Case study: Ann

Ann is a 20-year-old student studying diagnostic radiography. She enjoys her course and is doing well, but finds asking questions in class and making seminar presentations very difficult. Today, she has to do a five-minute talk, which she is dreading. She is surprised to find how dry her mouth has become, although her hands are sweaty. She has butterflies in her stomach and she is finding it difficult to concentrate on the preceding lectures. When she stands up to speak to the class, she shakes, her voice is higher than usual and she stammers slightly. Apart from this, she is enjoying student life, and has made some good friends. She is generally a quiet person who prefers concerts and the theatre to parties.

What is the matter with Ann? As you will have guessed, she is suffering from anxiety. You will almost certainly have experienced similar sensations at some time, perhaps before an examination. Anxiety is associated with the arousal of the autonomic nervous system and this gives rise to the physical symptoms described. Anxiety is a central issue in the study of psychology because of the debilitating effects it often has on people's lives and because psychological factors appear to be important causes. However, different models of psychology conceptualize and treat anxiety in different ways. Ann's problem will be examined using four psychological models and suggestions will be offered, based upon each of these models, for the management of her anxiety.

Exercise

Before you read any further, list all of the treatments for anxiety that you can think of or have heard of. If Ann went to her doctor and complained about her anxiety, what might he do?

Behaviourist approaches to dealing with Ann's anxiety

Behaviourism is the investigation of the way organisms learn, based upon observations of how they respond in different circumstances to different types of consequence. When Ann started her course, she found that everything seemed very strange, and rather frightening. However, after a while both the classroom and hospital environments became so familiar that she found it hard to understand how newcomers to these settings were feeling. This process is called **adaptation**. It allows us to focus our attention on new things in our environment without becoming overloaded with information.

One of the early behaviourists, John Watson, proposed that psychology should concentrate on observable behaviour and not concern itself with mental processes. He believed that learning was the basic foundation of all human activity and that if we could understand the process of learning, we would be able to develop universal laws which would predict behaviour. This is why psychologists set out to investigate the associations between stimuli (environmental events or changes) and behavioural responses. They could assess how behaviour was modified (or changed) by the experience of previous stimuli and responses. You will find a lot more detail about behaviourism and behaviourist theories in Chapter 4.

Behaviourists would not concern themselves with Ann's inner thoughts and feelings, but only with behaviour which an observer could record, the circumstances in which that behaviour occurs, and the immediate causes and consequences of the behaviour for the individual concerned.

Exercise

Ann exhibits a number of behaviours which indicate to an observer that she is anxious. List the observable behaviours which might indicate that an individual is anxious.

Behaviourists would probably argue that it is not necessary to know what originally caused Ann's anxiety in order to reduce or eliminate it. If pressed, they would probably explain Ann's anxiety in terms of her past experiences of speaking in public. There are two main behaviourist theories which may be used to account for this. The first is **classical conditioning**, in which a neutral or non-threatening stimulus (event or occurrence) triggers fear or anxiety because it has previously been associated with another aversive or threatening stimulus. This is based upon the work of Ivan Pavlov and John Watson early this century and you will find a more detailed account in Chapter 4. In the case of Ann's anxiety of speaking in public, this could have come about if a spider (the stimulus) had run up her leg as she stood up to ask a question in class at school one day, causing an intense fear response (assuming that she was frightened of spiders). One such occurrence could be sufficient to generate anxiety in similar future situations. In this case, her anxiety would be termed a **conditioned emotional response**.

The other main behaviourist theory is that of **operant conditioning**, which would suggest that her anxiety was caused by learning that speaking in public had unpleasant consequences. This explanation is based upon the **Law of effect**, described by Edward Thorndike at the beginning of this century, and later developed into a detailed account of the effects of **reinforcement** (positive consequences) and **punishment** (aversive consequences) on behaviour by B.F. Skinner. To illustrate this in Ann's case, she may have given incorrect answers to the teacher in class on a number of occasions. As a consequence of this, the other pupils may have laughed at her and mocked her. In this way, she would have found speaking in front of a group of other people an unpleasant and therefore anxiety-provoking experience, which she then tried to avoid.

If Ann went to a behavioural psychologist for treatment, the psychologist might not be too concerned about the original cause of her anxiety. Rather, they would concentrate on eliminating Ann's anxious behaviour. The assumption is that if Ann stops behaving as if she is anxious, then she no longer is anxious. Stop and think carefully about this. Can we assume, because someone looks and behaves as though they are confident and unconcerned, that they are not anxious?

There are a number of ways of treating anxiety, fears or phobias, using techniques which are derived from behaviourist psychology. In Ann's case, it is essential to ensure that she does not avoid public speaking altogether. She would undoubtedly avoid the source of her anxiety, but her inability to speak in public would not be cured. A popular approach, based upon the principles of classical conditioning, is that of **systematic desensitization**, developed by Joseph Wolpe in the late 1950s. The psychologist would first teach Ann relaxation skills because it is impossible to relax and be tense at the same time. Then she would be asked to imagine speaking to a small group of friends while rehearsing her relaxation skills. During her programme of treatment, she would practise relaxation while gradually working through speaking to a small formal group and then to larger groups, first in her imagination and then in reality, until her anxiety had subsided sufficiently to allow her to relax while addressing a large group. In this way, public speaking ceases to be an anxiety-provoking task. This approach would be equally appropriate for treating Ann's fear of spiders.

Another approach, based upon operant conditioning, would be to ensure that all members of the class are asked to give regular short presentations in the relative safety of their class environment and that the rest of the class are expected to give encouraging (as opposed to critical) feedback to Ann. This would ensure that Ann is eventually able to associate public speaking with positive reinforcing, rather than negative punishing consequences, thus allowing her anxious behaviours to be eliminated.

Exercise

Think of something that you feel apprehensive about. Plan how you might use behavioural principles to help you to tackle this.

Cognitive approaches to Ann's anxiety

An alternative approach to understanding people's behaviour is to consider their cognitive (thought) processes. Cognitive psychologists are concerned primarily with thought processes (i.e. **cognition**), including perception (how we sense and interpret what is going on around us), learning and memory, intelligence and language. Psychophysiologists would be interested in how these processes are linked to brain activity. For example, they may use electroencephalograms (EEG) to record changes in brain waves when people are trying to learn something new. Cognitive psychologists tend to use abstract models which enable them to understand how these processes occur, without worrying too much about identifying specific neural pathways. They have recently become interested in artificial intelligence and computerized models of human information processing. In this book, we have chosen to concentrate on the cognitive areas of learning, perception and memory, which are to be found in Chapters 4 and 5, since these are of most direct relevance to health care. Readers who are interested in issues relating to intelligence, language and information processing are directed to general psychology texts, such as Gross (1992) and Atkinson *et al.* (1993), or to other texts which deal with these specific topics.

In Ann's case, we can assume that she is of adequate intelligence, since she has been accepted for her undergraduate course on the basis of her educational qualifications. She has a good command of the English language and this is not the cause of her problem. However, someone who normally stutters badly, or who has a problem with the pronunciation of certain sounds, or even someone who is embarrassed about their regional accent, might feel anxious about revealing these in public. If Ann's problem was related to a speech difficulty, then speech therapy or assertiveness training might represent possible solutions, depending upon the nature of the problem.

Assuming that Ann's anxiety is related to the situation (public speaking), rather than the means of communication, the cognitive psychologist might, like the behavioural psychologist, explain the cause in terms of her past experiences. However, unlike behavioural psychologists, a cognitive psychologist would be interested in finding out how Ann interprets her problem. They would use her interpretation as the basis for changing the way she thinks about it, on the assumption that this will change her behaviour.

Suppose that Ann believes that her fear of public speaking relates back to her experiences of ridicule in the classroom. This would mean that every time she stands up to speak, she is reliving her past humiliation and is expecting that her presentation will, once again, lead to embarrassment. The cognitive psychologist would help her to reinterpret her past experiences in more positive terms. This approach is termed **cognitive therapy**. An alternative explanation for her past experiences might be that her classmates had laughed because they were relieved that it was her, rather than themselves, who was asked those questions. Therefore, they were not laughing at her, but letting go of their own tension. This type of explanation would enable Ann to think about her current situation in a different and more positive way, and encourage her to rehearse positive and reassuring self-talk before standing up. In this way, the negative experience of public speaking becomes reinterpreted as a positive one and this builds up confidence. Using this approach, it is possible to reduce anxiety by mental preparation for a feared activity, and to make a more positive realistic interpretation of the activity so that it is perceived to be less threatening.

There are other possible cognitive explanations for anxiety about speaking in public. It may be that Ann has had difficulty in remembering the facts and figures necessary to answer questions. Memory processes and their application in health care are covered in Chapter 5. Some people think that their memory is worse than others, but most of us are capable of improving our memory through the use of memory-enhancing techniques. If Ann is asked to give a presentation to the class, she will be well advised to prepare it thoroughly and write out a series of prompt cards, or give key points on acetates used on the overhead projector, if she does not wish to read out the whole script.

The psychodynamic approach

The psychodynamic approach to psychological problems has its origins with Freud and **psychoanalysis**. Freud's ideas have had a tremendous influence on the ways in which lay people think and talk about motivations and unconscious processes. People commonly use Freudian terms and concepts like denial, repression and ego in everyday conversation without even realizing it. Freud's ideas have been developed and used by a number of health care disciplines over the last century. Freud has made a contribution to psychological debate in the areas of personality, development, motivation, the unconscious and treatment for mental health problems. Psychoanalysis is a method of inquiry, a theory of mind and a mode of treatment.

Sigmund Freud was born in 1856. By the turn of the century, he was a medical doctor specializing in neurology in Vienna. He discovered that some patients had physical problems which appeared to result from previous emotional trauma. He wrote a description of one of his early patients, Anna O, who consulted Freud and his colleagues because she had a paralysis of her arm. There seemed to be no neurological reason for this, but by talking to her and using hypnosis, Freud identified the likely origin of her problems as psychological. Anna had cared for her father at home when he was dying. She used to sit by his bed all night. One night she fell asleep with her arm over the back of her chair and when she woke up her arm had 'pins and needles' and felt numb. So great was her alarm that her arm became useless to her. Freud called this condition 'conversion hysteria' (a psychological fear which is converted into a physical or somatic problem). Freud found that by getting such patients to relive their experiences and their emotions, they were sometimes cured. He called this discharge of emotions **catharsis**.

Psychoanalytic psychotherapists (more usually referred to these days as psychodynamic psychotherapists) mainly treat patients who have emotional problems, such as severe anxiety or depression. They now rarely use the psychoanalyst's couch, but they still use a therapy which is based upon talking about salient memories and past experiences, particularly those which occurred in early childhood and which may have been repressed. *Repression* is not a conscious process but a mechanism by which the ego protects itself from threatening events. The individual might be asked to describe dreams or make spontaneous word associations. It is thought that these emerge from the subconscious to reveal repressed experiences and allow catharsis to occur. New interpretations of repressed experiences, with the aid of the therapist, help people make quite major changes to the way they understand themselves and their relationships.

One of the problems with using this approach is that there is a wide range of possible explanations for Ann's anxiety. To attribute her anxiety to an incident or even a series of incidents in school might be regarded as too simplistic. According to Freud, anxiety is an unpleasant state which is caused by tension between the *id* (the most basic part of the personality involved in the satisfaction of basic instincts such as food and sex), the *ego* (that part of the personality which balances the fulfilment of these basic instincts with what is socially acceptable) and the *superego* (the social conscience). According to Freud, the ego develops during childhood as the child passes through certain stages of development: first, the oral stage, in which the baby obtains pleasure from sucking; second, the anal stage, in which the focus is on toilet training and the child can choose to give or withhold faeces in order to provide pleasure, or to please or annoy the mother; third, the phallic stage, in which pleasure is gained from the genitalia. There is then a latency period before the genital stage of adult development is reached at puberty.

These stages have been much simplified here. However, Freud described how development may be arrested at any stage. For example, if Ann smoked heavily to control her anxiety, this might suggest that her development had been arrested at the oral stage because she likes to have something constantly in her mouth. One of the purposes of psychodynamic psychotherapy in this case would be to assist her to progress through the remaining stages of development by working through certain aspects of her childhood which are unresolved. The relationship with her mother and father would be a central feature of therapy. Freud proposed that during the phallic stage of development (at about 4–6 years of age), boys fantasize about their mothers (the Oedipus complex) while girls fantasize about their fathers. The latter idea appears to have emerged from Freud's contact with a predominantly female client population, a number of whom claimed to have been sexually abused as children by their fathers. Nowadays, we might be more inclined to believe these reports than assign them to the realms of fantasy.

According to a psychoanalytic view, Ann's anxiety may not be cured until she has come to terms with, and worked through, problems with her relationship with her parents. Perhaps she had always had difficulty in 'speaking up' for herself at home and at school. Maybe her mother had a traditional role in the family and was unable to stand up to her husband. The psychotherapist would help Ann to gain insight into the origins of her anxiety and help her to change her responses. An example of an analysis undertaken by Freud is given in Gross (1994, ch. 20) and the reader may find it useful to consult this.

Psychoanalysis can be a lengthy process, and those who engage in this form of psychotherapy frequently remain in therapy for years. They often get better and attribute this to the therapy. However, most people manage to overcome all sorts of problems in their lives as their circumstances change and they learn new or alternative ways of coping with different situations. If Ann eventually overcame her difficulties with public speaking after six months of therapy, it would be difficult to know if it was the therapy which was responsible for this, or if it was due to an entirely different set of factors.

> **Exercise**
>
> Can you think of any problems which might arise if health professionals use a psychoanalytic approach to analyse patients' problems, without the benefit of specialist training? Find out what sort of training is required to practise as a psychoanalytic or psychodynamic psychologist.

Since Freud's death, other psychologists have modified certain aspects of psychoanalytic theory. However, the basic belief that anxiety disorders have their origins in individual development remains a fundamental tenet of the psychodynamic approach to psychotherapy. One of the main problems with taking a psychodynamic view of Ann's anxiety is that the focus is often primarily on individual unconscious processes, rather than on situational causes. Ann's difficulty might be taken to indicate that she has a neurotic personality and is therefore anxiety-prone, when in fact she is only anxious in specific situations like public speaking. A psychotherapist would be unlikely to make this mistake; however, this type of labelling is not uncommon when health care professionals make lay use of psychological concepts. It can lead to some unfortunate consequences for patients, some of which are considered in Chapter 9.

People have tried, without much success, to test Freud's theories experimentally, and there is much controversy over the current status of psychoanalytic theory within psychology. Critics point out that such a global and all-encompassing explanation of humanity is very difficult to falsify and it does not, therefore, satisfy the demands of a sound scientific theory. Furthermore, psychoanalytic interpretations tend to be subjective, thus leaving their validity open to question. Overall, psychoanalysis remains controversial for many psychologists and non-psychologists.

Humanistic approaches

Humanistic psychology has its origins in existentialism and phenomenology, in which causal explanations are of relatively little interest. The phenomenological approach to psychology tries to understand each individual's unique world view, or perspective. These world views are part of our taken-for-granted way of seeing the world. Without some careful reflection, it is difficult to be aware of our own individual way of seeing the world.

The focus of humanistic psychology is on the here and now, on the concept of the self and how I feel about myself. In fact, the importance of the 'self' as a separate part of the person, distinct from social and family relationships, is a very Western notion. Some cultures (e.g. China and the Islamic countries) emphasize the collective nature of human beings and their embeddedness in social contexts. In Britain and the United States, individual success is seen in terms of obtaining a good job and earning a lot of money, rather than maintaining and reciprocating in long-term relationships. This may be one of the many reasons for the increasing divorce rate.

Carl Rogers is the humanistic psychologist most commonly associated with the theory of the self. He worked with people who had emotional problems but rejected both the behaviourist and psychoanalytic approaches which were prevalent in the 1950s. Instead, he explored individuals' subjective understanding of their 'self'. This is the 'I' or 'me' that I currently conceptualize myself as being. Many of us actually have great difficulty in knowing and understanding who we really are and, for some, finding themselves has become an important preoccupation. The **self concept** can be defined as the way one thinks about one's self. In reality, the self concept is not fixed but is in a constant state of flux. I can be confident one minute and uncertain the next; feel good about myself in one situation and totally worthless in another. Rogers (see Thorne 1992) described how some people have faith in their own judgement, while others tend to turn to others for reassurance and self-evaluation. Most people are motivated by the approval from others. Rogers referred to this as the need for positive regard.

Rogers introduced the concept of **self-actualization**. He conceptualized this as an innate tendency which drives all individuals to achieve their full potential, within the limits of environmental or situational constraints. Rogers noted that people who came to him with psychological problems exhibited a natural tendency towards growth and maturity which enabled them to overcome many of their own problems. According to Rogers, psychological problems have their origins in childhood, when love and acceptance are made conditional upon performance and achievement. He suggested that personal growth is best achieved in an atmosphere of **unconditional positive regard**, in which the parent accepts the child for what he or she is, and not what the parent would like him or her to be. Conditional love builds up a conflict within the child between the self, as they perceive themselves to be, and the self that they would like to be. This leads to low **self-esteem** (feelings of self-worth). In the case of Ann, her anxiety may have been engendered by her perceived failure to meet the high standards of public behaviour demanded by her parents. This may have made her frightened to make any type of public appearance or statement for fear of their disapproval.

Rogers believed that, given the freedom and opportunity, people can spontaneously reveal their own concerns and often have sufficient insight to identify their own solutions to problems. The type of therapy associated with Rogers is **Rogerian counselling** or *client-centred therapy*, which is currently growing in popularity in primary care. Rogerian counsellors are non-judgemental, non-directive, and display warmth, empathy and personal regard for their clients. Counselling is quite different from psychoanalysis in that the therapist makes no attempt to interpret the client's problems or direct a course of action. It is a technique which has become very popular with nurses and midwives, although it is rare for counselling sessions to be truly non-directive.

A humanistic approach to Ann's problems might involve her attending a student counselling service. The counsellor would give Ann the opportunity to talk through her fears of being humiliated in class. As she talked, she might start to gain personal insight into her problems, identify her own solutions and feel good about herself in the process. The counsellor would encourage her to value herself for what she is and not to strive to be something she is not. Once she feels better about herself, she will not worry so much about what other people think about her. She may then feel able to stand up in class with more self-confidence.

Exercise

Do you think that non-directive counselling is likely to be appropriate for every sort of person and every type of problem? Discuss this with other members of your group. What sort of people do you think might benefit most from non-directive counselling? What types of problem are unlikely to be amenable to counselling? (You may wish to return to this exercise once you have read about other aspects of psychology in Chapters 3, 4 and 6.)

An important way in which we develop our own sense of ourselves is by comparing ourselves with other people and building up an image of what we would like to be. George Kelly, the originator of **personal construct theory** (see Chapter 5), was a psychologist working within the humanistic tradition who devised a way of identifying important individual comparisons through the use of a **repertory grid**. In the case of Ann, she would be invited to select important people in her life (significant others). She would then be asked to identify the ways in which these people are the same and the ways in which they are different from herself, using her own **bipolar** (positive *vs* negative) descriptions (e.g. tall/short). She would also identify how she perceives herself to be (her **actual self**), and the self she would like to be (her **ideal self**). The resulting grid might look something like Fig. 1.1.

A grid like this might indicate that Ann had grown up comparing herself to an older sister who was clever, attractive and outgoing. She may, as a result, feel inferior in all of these respects. She may also see her best friend as more intelligent and attractive than herself. In view of her progress on her course and her ability to make friends, she probably has unrealistically negative views of herself and low self-esteem. A therapist who uses a personal construct approach might encourage Ann to identify ways in which she would like to improve. The therapist might encourage her

	Myself as I am	Myself as I would like to be	Older sister	Best friend
Intelligent (√) Dull (×)	×	√	√	√
Attractive (√) Plain (×)	×	√	√	√
Outgoing (√) Shy (×)	×	√	√	×

Figure 1.1 Repertory grid showing positive and negative comparisons between Ann and significant others.

to develop and rehearse a new characterization or role in the safety of the therapeutic environment. This might be directed towards giving a confident presentation and would give her more confidence in real-life classroom situations.

While Rogers conceptualized self-actualization as a process, Abraham Maslow (1970) described it as the epitome of achievement, to be obtained once all other more basic needs had been fulfilled. He based this on reports of interviews with people whom he judged to have reached their full potential, including Albert Einstein and Abraham Lincoln. The characteristics of this concept include acceptance of self and others for what they are (no discrepancy between actual and ideal self and no consistent discrepancy between self and others); the ability to tolerate uncertainty; creativity; the use of problem-centred rather than self-centred approaches to dealing with issues; and strong moral and ethical standards.

Maslow was first and foremost an experimental psychologist who had worked within both the behaviourist and psychoanalytic schools of psychology before adopting a phenomenological approach to understanding the human condition. He incorporated the concept of self-actualization into his '**hierarchy of needs**', which is illustrated in Fig. 1.2. His model of human needs is based upon observations in different cultures. This has provided the basis of many needs-based models of nursing (e.g. Roper, Logan and Tierney) and has proved popular with other professions involved in caring for, or working with, people. It has proved less popular with other psychologists, perhaps because it is difficult to support with objective research findings. The hierarchy is part of a theory which proposes that lower-order needs must be met before higher-order needs can be fulfilled. Self-actualization represents the pinnacle in the realization of personal achievement.

In Ann's case, it is possible that her needs for esteem have not yet been met. This may impede her academic progress and a Rogerian counsellor might seek to improve Ann's self-esteem to enable her to maximize her potential on her course.

The evaluation of humanistic theories rather depends upon your particular world view. If you perceive scientific validation (in terms of

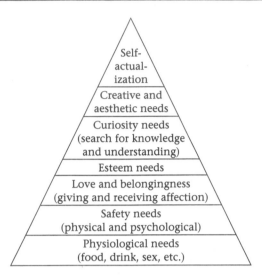

Figure 1.2   Maslow's hierarchy of needs (adapted from Maslow 1970).

Exercise

Write down where you think you lie on Maslow's hierarchy. How far are you from reaching a state of self-actualization? Have you ever had what might be described as a 'peak experience'? If so, under what circumstances? What needs do you need to fulfil in order to move higher up the hierarchy? How might you achieve this? How easy is it to judge where you are at present?

experimental support) as important, then 'self' theories do not fulfil these requirements. However, they are intuitively appealing. The theories are valuable for health professionals because they emphasize how important it is to realize that a problem like anxiety is likely to be experienced by different individuals in very different ways. In addition, these theories provide an optimistic non-pathologizing account of human beings. We are not to be seen as merely victims of our genes, early learning experiences, or instincts, but that we are all able to develop until we feel that we have reached our full potential. These issues are developed further in Chapter 3. The need to listen to people and provide them with opportunities to disclose worries and concerns has become very popular in health care, and counselling skills are currently being taught on many courses.

Other approaches to understanding psychological problems

This chapter has introduced four common approaches used by psychologists to understand human beings with particular reference to anxiety. These were selected because they provide contrasting ways of conceptualizing an important common psychological issue. By now, you will have recognized that these approaches have some similarities but a lot of differences. Some actually conflict with each other in terms of their interpretations and their therapeutic approaches. Attempts to identify which approach is most effective have proved problematic, since few therapists adopt a purist approach. Many combine aspects of different therapies into what is termed an **eclectic** approach. Research indicates that therapies which use a focused approach (including cognitive–behavioural therapies) are associated with better outcomes (Shapiro and Shapiro 1982), while counselling is probably the most popular approach for relatively minor problems. It is likely that, in reality, patients select the therapist with whom they have a rapport and the therapy which best suits their individual coping style (see Chapter 6).

One treatment which was not considered above, but which would have been the most common method of treatment had Ann consulted her doctor up until a few years ago, is the prescription of tranquillizers. This is based upon a medical model which conceptualizes anxiety as an abnormal physiological response. Tranquillizers were once seen as the answer to a variety of psychological problems, since they reduced some of the physiological symptoms of anxiety. Psychologists have long argued that this was not treating the actual problem. However, it took the identification of problems of drug-dependence and **iatrogenesis** (medically induced side-effects or illnesses) to stop wholesale prescribing. Even now, new wonder drugs or 'happy pills' are being pushed by their manufacturers as the answer to the common and frequently disabling psychological problems of anxiety and depression. You are invited to use this book to decide for yourselves about the wisdom of such an approach.

Other important psychological ways of focusing on people are covered later in this book, and can be found in other texts. Psychophysiologists studying stress are interested in how the body reacts in terms of both mental and physical changes. They study the interaction of psychological processes with physiological mechanisms, such as autonomic responses, blood pressure control and immune system functioning, and measure neurological, hormonal and immunological responses alongside self-reports of feelings and sensations such as anxiety. In the example of Ann, they might be interested in studying how her feelings of anxiety, dry mouth and sweaty hands are associated with measurable physiological changes. They might ask questions like, 'Which change came first, the subjective perception of anxiety or the physical changes?' Over the longer term, they might want to investigate whether chronic anxiety would lead to permanent physiological changes and cause conditions such as hypertension (high blood pressure). The interrelationship between psychological and physiological processes is termed **psychosomatic**. A psychosomatic disorder is one which involves both physical and psychological components, although it does *not* imply that one causes the other. Pain is a good example of this and is examined in some detail in Chapter 8.

A set of theories not addressed in this book are trait theories of personality, of which there are many. Many of you will be familiar with the terms 'introvert', 'extrovert', 'neurotic' and 'psychotic', which were

developed by trait theorists, including Hans Eysenck, to describe relatively
stable personality characteristics. While these may be of interest to those
who wish to extend their knowledge of psychology, this book cannot
cover every aspect in depth, and the decision to omit these relates to their
limited utility for health care professionals at this level. Personality traits
often provide a convenient label, but tell us little about applications in
health care and are often misinterpreted by those who engage in 'pop'
psychology. To describe Ann (or anyone else for that matter) as a neurotic
introvert (often loosely translated as an unstable loner who worries a lot)
serves no useful purpose for any health care professional, since it provides
no indication about how Ann's problem can be managed. In fact, these
labels are often used as an excuse for doing nothing.

Another important area of individual differences which will not be
addressed here is the issue of intelligence. The nature–nurture debate [the
extent to which standardized intelligence quotient (IQ) levels are a
consequence of our genes or our upbringing] is still an issue in the 1990s.
Although there is plenty of evidence to suggest that each interacts with
the other to determine intellectual achievement, the balance between the
two factors is still hotly contended. Of course, these issues have important
implications for race relations, since any suggestion of innate differences
may lead to discrimination. Many people probably fail to achieve their
full potential because of low expectations and may be a self-fulfilling
prophecy. Ann appears to provide a good example of having low expectations of oneself.

Another major perspective in psychology, which will be examined in
relation to health issues in Chapter 7, is the developmental approach.
Psychologists are interested in the whole lifespan of a person from the
very first social relationships formed between a baby and its parents, to
what happens in old age when friends and family die and these relationships
are lost. There is a developmental perspective to almost every aspect of
human functioning; for example, how much a newborn baby is able to
see, and how children learn language. These and many more questions
have been asked (and occasionally answered) by psychologists. One of the
central debates in this area, as in intelligence, is the extent to which
development is influenced by genetic inheritance as opposed to environmental influences, such as the type of schooling, the 'warmth' of parenting
experienced, and the culture in which the person is reared. If it was
possible to provide such a detailed analysis of Ann's development, it might
be possible to trace her lack of self-esteem to an interaction between her
genetic make-up, which may have imbued her with a sense of uncertainty
about interpreting her surroundings, and an upbringing which failed to
provide the consistency and security necessary to accommodate this. As
it is, we can only make inferences about her past.

Finally, a key area of psychology for health care professionals, which
sometimes overlaps with sociology, is social psychology. All humans, and
many other animals, live in complex social systems. The health service is
an example of a complex organization where many different people are
required to work together in multidisciplinary teams. We are all influenced
by our interaction with other people, including colleagues, patients and
their families. Social psychology has relevance to every aspect of our daily

lives, our interactions with others and the way we interpret and learn about events. Chapter 9 will explore these social processes and examine their relevance to the delivery of health care.

What is a psychologist?

The difference between a psychiatrist and a psychologist

The final section of this chapter is designed to assist in identifying the different professionals and types of psychologist who are involved in health care and the delivery of health care services.

A psychiatrist is someone who has qualified as a medical doctor and then specializes in the diagnosis and treatment of people with mental health disorders. They tend (but not always) to have an organic view of mental health problems. They commonly use a range of therapies, often including drug treatments, and sometimes use physical interventions like the controversial electroconvulsive therapy (ECT). In comparison, a psychologist will have completed a first degree, in which psychology was the major component, and then taken a further specialist educational programme (e.g. clinical, education and occupational psychology). These psychologists are concerned not only with assessing and helping individuals, but with advising groups and organizations. In addition to academic and research psychologists, applied psychologists are to be found working in such fields as road transport research, criminal psychology and information technology. Health psychology is a recent applied field of psychology which is concerned with research into the promotion of health and quality of life, the prevention of illness and rehabilitation processes.

Educational psychologists

Educational psychologists generally work in schools and are qualified teachers as well as specialist psychologists. They are involved in the assessment of children who have special educational needs. Based upon their detailed assessment, the psychologist provides a 'statement' which describes the help and resources that the child requires. For example, some children (commonly boys) experience great difficulty in concentrating in class. They may frequently get up and move around during lessons, and may be disruptive by talking or shouting. These children are sometimes labelled 'hyperactive'. Their behaviour disrupts the teacher and other children's attention, and it also means that the child is punished a lot but receives little education. Psychologists have developed special learning programmes for these children, and work with their teachers and parents to achieve better control of the child's behaviour.

Occupational psychologists

Occupational psychology involves understanding how people function at work. Occupational psychologists may advise on selection procedures where they often use psychological tests to identify features such as aptitude and honesty. They also study the workplace environment. For example, they may be brought in to advise on how patients' monitors and alarms can best be arranged in highly technical areas like intensive care units (ICUs). They also advise on organizational management and the management of change, which is now a core element of education at all levels for health care professionals.

You may be interested to know that much research has investigated occupational stress in nurses and other health professionals, including the effects of working shifts. The field of health care is recognized to be very stressful and a knowledge of organizational factors in stress management can be very helpful to all health care professionals. This is addressed towards the end of Chapter 6.

Clinical psychologists

Practising clinical psychologists may be based in hospitals, in general practitioner (GP) surgeries, in community clinics or in private practice. They will have spent three years undertaking additional education in the assessment, care, treatment and prevention of mental health disorders. Clinical psychologists use a range of approaches to help clients. Most of them specialize in working with particular groups, like elderly people, people with learning difficulties, or those with acute or chronic mental health problems. For example, a clinical psychologist might be part of a multidisciplinary team working with drug-using adolescents. They would be able to contribute their special knowledge about normal teenage development, processes of addiction, behavioural therapeutic techniques and counselling skills. Clinical psychologists like to describe themselves as scientist-practitioners. In other words, they are keen to apply psychological theories and research in helping their clients. Recently, they have become more involved in helping people with physical illness, and also in designing and implementing preventative and rehabilitative programmes, for example in heart disease. Finally, some clinical psychologists have a role in providing staff support and in teaching stress management skills.

Health psychologists

Health psychologists have only recently emerged as a distinct group. They usually have a higher degree in health psychology, which, unlike one in clinical psychology, is not practice-based. In reality, many health psychologists are either clinical psychologists or health professionals with a higher degree in health psychology. They have specialist knowledge of the factors which influence health behaviour change in primary, secondary and tertiary prevention, stress and stress management, and communication issues in health care. They usually apply their knowledge through research or consultancy but, unlike clinical psychologists, are not involved in implementing individual treatment programmes. It is perhaps no coincidence that health psychology has assumed importance at a time when there is increasing emphasis upon the need to promote effective health behaviour change through health promotion and education.

Summary

- Psychology is the study of behaviour and mental processes.
- The study of psychology is important to understand people we work with and ourselves.
- It is important to understand the ideas and principles of psychology so that they may be interpreted and applied correctly.
- Chapter 1 has introduced four main approaches:
  - behaviourism,
  - cognitive psychology,
  - psychodynamic theories,
  - humanistic perspectives on the 'self'.
- Physiological, developmental and social approaches are also used in the application of psychological principles.
- Different types of psychologist work in various health care services and settings.

Further reading

Any introductory textbook in psychology will provide more detail about the approaches presented in this chapter.

Atkinson, R.L., Atkinson, R.C., Smith, E.E. and Bem, D.J. (1993) *Introduction to Psychology*, 11th edn. Orlando, FL: Harcourt Brace Jovanovich.

Bernstein, D.A., Clarke-Stewart, A., Roy, E.J., Srull, T.K. and Wickens, C.D. (1994) *Psychology*, 3rd edn. Boston, MA: Houghton Mifflin. Chapters 1 and 2.

Gross R.D. (1992) *Psychology: The Science of Mind and Behaviour*, 2nd edn. London: Hodder and Stoughton.

Hayes, N. (1994) *Foundations of Psychology*. London: Routledge. Chapter 1.

CHAPTER TWO

UNDERSTANDING HEALTH AND ILLNESS

Introduction

'Can a person have a disease but feel healthy?' 'Can a person feel ill but have no disease?' 'How do people make decisions about health care behaviours like screening?' This chapter will examine these and other questions concerning how people understand being healthy and being ill. Lay (as opposed to health professional) representations of illness are considered, together with the influence of cultural factors on these attributions. Examples of cross-cultural research will be used to illustrate differences in the recognition of disease and attributions about causation. The second part of the chapter will focus on psychological models which attempt to predict health-related behaviours. The assumptions that underpin these models are discussed and their relevance to health care evaluated.

Disease and illness

In Western societies, the medical model has been the main model of health and illness this century. The medical model focuses upon patterns of organic pathology which are termed diseases. For example, diabetes can be identified in relation to certain specific biochemical evidence, such as raised blood sugar levels. Diseases are actually abstract things, but are assumed to be identical wherever they occur. Diabetes, whether in Britain or Papua New Guinea, is assumed to be the same entity. The medical model takes no account of the meaning people give to the disease nor how they cope with it. In comparison, illness refers to the subjective experience of disease. It depends on the meaning that a person places on a set of symptoms. To summarize, a disease is something an organ has, while illness is something a person has. Within the medical model, health has traditionally been conceptualized as the absence of disease.

Theoretical perspectives

Anthropologists, sociologists and psychologists have conceptualized health and illness in rather different ways. These are examined below in order to provide a context for understanding what is meant by health and illness.

Anthropological perspectives

Anthropology is the study of people within their cultural groups. In the early part of this century, people and cultures were thought of as being divided into those which were 'civilized' and those which were 'primitive'. Western biomedicine was regarded as objective and rational when compared with primitive medicine which was based on magic, ritual and religion. This view is now seen to be very judgemental and ethnocentric. Anthropologists now propose that medical systems develop from the cultural beliefs within a society and can only be understood within the context of these belief systems, so Western medicine is regarded as just one system among many others. Moreover, within a society there are likely to be a range of health beliefs. For example, in Britain, people may use complementary treatments, orthodox medical therapies and their own home remedies, although each therapy may be based on rather different beliefs about the causes of the illness. It is interesting how practitioners of biomedicine have attempted to discredit other views by labelling other healers or practitioners, including homeopaths, as 'quacks'. Kleinman (1980) suggests that cultures provide people with ways of thinking about symptoms. This enables them to determine which problems can be defined as illness and what should be done about them.

FOCUS ON	**'High-pertension': A folk model of illness**
RESEARCH	Hypertension is a serious condition in which both diastolic and systolic blood pressure remain consistently raised. This may lead to potentially serious consequences such as stroke and renal disease. Unfortunately, the condition is asymptomatic, so it is difficult for

people to know when their blood pressure is high without it being measured. In Western medicine, drug treatment is used to reduce blood pressure, but there are a number of unpleasant side-effects from the medication. An anthropological study investigated the beliefs of 60 elderly African-American women living in New Orleans (Heurtin-Roberts 1993). These women differentiated between two conditions, high blood and high-pertension. They thought that high blood was a permanent 'disease of the blood and heart' (p. 288), caused by eating the wrong (fatty) foods, heredity and to a lesser extent stress, and that it was treatable by anti-hypertensive medication. In comparison, high-pertension was seen as a more transient 'disease of the nerves' caused by stress, worry and anger. The women perceived a structural model of the condition in which, during episodes of stress, the blood would rise up in the body to the head. They could recall particular stressful times in their lives which had resulted in high-pertension. Treatment concerned reducing stress by withdrawing from people or relaxing, rather than taking medication. High-pertension was seen to result from their interactions with a hostile environment. Many respondents were poor, living in inadequate housing and having low-paid employment. Heurtin-Roberts argued that high-pertension was an expression of distress in the social conditions in which these women found themselves. One women said:

> There's a lot of high blood pressure in my family. I'm the only one with high-pertension though. High blood is something you inherit, but high-pertension comes from nerves. It got bad as I got older. I guess you have more problems as you get older.

Sociological perspectives

Early medical sociologists viewed Western biomedicine as benign and emphasized its functional role in caring for the sick. Parsons (1951) described the 'sick role' in terms of rights and obligations.

Sick people have the right to:

- withdraw from their normal social roles
- be cared for

and an obligation to:

- follow medical advice
- get better as soon as possible.

Subsequent theorists were more critical of Western medicine and focused in particular upon the power relationships within society and medicine. For example, Illich (1976) wrote a major critique of American medical institutions which, he thought, had a pathologizing impact on daily life. There has been a trend for social problems, or even normal life events like childbirth, the menopause and dying, to be redefined as medical concerns. This can have mixed results. For example, it could result in a hyperactive child being sent for medical treatment rather than being beaten in school. However, this also results in the child being labelled as psychiatrically ill and perhaps being prescribed long-term medication, while in the past the child would have just been labelled bad. Zola (1972) has described four ways in which our everyday lives have become medicalized:

- Medicalization of private lives – we are bombarded with advice on eating, exercise and sexual behaviour
- Medical influence in public life – for example, the compulsory use of seat-belts in cars, the banning of smoking on public transport
- Medical control over procedures like prescribing drugs or gaining access to specialist services
- Medical dominance in 'taboo' areas such as child abuse

> ### Exercise: Health advice
>
> Select a newspaper or women's magazine. Carefully note down all the health advice given. You may prefer to group these into topics, such as diet, exercise, stress reduction, etc. What types of advice are given? What recommendations are made? What assumptions underlie this advice? Is any of the advice contradictory? How much notice do you think people take of this advice?

An alternative sociological perspective focuses upon social constructionist theories which emphasize the role people play in finding and thinking up explanations for illness. The term 'hyperactive' is essentially a label which is used to describe very active, fidgety children who lack concentration. Placing a label such as this on a set of symptoms is meaningful, since it determines our own, and other people's, subsequent behaviours and attitudes. In the case of hyperactivity, it may remove guilt from the parents who are able to justify their child's behaviour in terms of illness, rather than a result of poor parental discipline. Over the years, societies have changed their views about what is regarded as an illness. Some famous examples from the past are drapetomania (which was the term used to describe the tendency of slaves to run away) or homosexual behaviour. Neither of these would be termed an 'illness' in the 1990s. However, we have relatively new conditions like premenstrual tension (PMT) or the 'male menopause'. What are the advantages and disadvantages of diagnoses like these?

It seems that defining health and illness is not a simple matter of being right or wrong in biomedical terms. People have available to them a range of explanations which they choose to make use of. At the moment, you are probably learning biomedical theories of disease causation, but you will also be aware of lay theories (also called folk models) which were used within your own family to explain disease. We are often unaware of our taken-for-granted theories of illness.

Exercise

What does being healthy mean? Why are you healthy? Write down all the reasons you can think of. Ask other people, including your mother and your grandmother. Do the lists vary? Why might this be?

Stainton Rogers (1991) investigated explanations of health and illness provided by British adults. She grouped them into eight separate categories:

1 *The body as a machine account.* Illness is seen as a malfunction which the doctor (the mechanic) needs to fix, for example by replacement surgery.
2 *The body under siege account.* People feel threatened by the environment (pollution), the stress of modern life and germs. For example, some people blame air pollution for asthma.
3 *The inequality of access account.* This focuses on the unequal distribution of resources and health care services. A current concern is whether GPs who are 'fund-holders' (manage their own budgets) are able to get better and quicker access to hospital services for their patients, compared with other doctors.
4 *The cultural critique of medicine.* This view is derived from sociological models which emphasize the role of power and oppression in society. Feminist writers like Ann Oakley have demonstrated how medical services for pregnant women can fail to value their experiences as mothers because 'expert' knowledge of pregnancy and childbirth is seen to be the domain of obstetricians.
5 *The health promotion account.* This was the message advocated by the government's *Health of the Nation* document (DoH 1992a), that healthy lifestyles prevent disease. People are urged to make 'healthy choices', although little regard is given to situational constraints, such as the cost of fresh fruit and vegetables.
6 *The robust individualism account.* This perspective regards the rights of individuals as more important than fear of disease. It is an argument used by smokers who oppose personal restriction on their 'liberty' to smoke in public places.
7 *The God's power account.* This views health in terms of spiritual well-being and being under God's protection. This position suggests that prayer or faith are important components of healing.
8 *The willpower account.* This is an individualistic view of health which stresses the moral responsibility of people to maintain their health. It becomes a controversial issue in health care when doctors refuse to treat patients with heart disease who refuse to stop smoking.

You may want to compare some of these explanations to the attributions you found in the last exercise. A further study by Furnham (1994) developed a questionnaire from these eight accounts and found that people generally believe that their health is influenced by psychological attributes and well-being, access to health services, their employment and living conditions, societal or cultural issues, and fate and religious factors.

Lay understanding of illness

How do people make sense of symptoms? Helman (1978) suggested that people ask themselves a series of questions:

- What has happened?
- Why has it happened?
- Why to me?
- Why now?
- What would happen if nothing was done about it?
- What should I do about it?
- Whom should I consult for further help?

Consider a common symptom like a headache and think about what might be the processes involved in understanding the meaning of a head-ache. The interpretation of symptoms is derived from internal sensations, information from the social environment, such as what others think, and information based on past experiences of headache and illness. First, you have to be aware of physiological changes such as a throbbing feeling in the head. This needs to reach a certain critical level and persist for a time before you become aware of it. The symptom then becomes labelled and acknowledged, and a search made for the reasons for it. You might be able to dismiss the throbbing as only to be expected if you were at the time sitting in a noisy power boat. You might also attribute the throbbing to loud noise at a disco and not define yourself as being ill at all but as having a good time. However, if you are sitting at home and your head is throbbing, you might consider what to do next. You may decide to do nothing because you know from past experience that headaches pass off in time, or you may take a couple of aspirin tablets. Your cures are likely to be selected on the basis of the **causal attributions** you make (the most likely reasons): fresh air for too much smoking; a long relaxing bath for a tension headache; and so on. Of course, if the headache is very severe or lasts a long time, you may become worried. Indeed, worrying might make your headache worse. You may compare your headache with previous ones, or with the headaches other people report. Of course, we can never really know how bad other people's symptoms are, which makes such comparison processes very difficult. At the next stage, you may ask family or friends for advice, then take a trip to the pharmacist to buy stronger medication before seeking medical help. By the time people arrive in hospital, they have been through a long process of thinking about and trying to understand their symptoms. However, their attributions and their understanding may be quite different from our medical interpretation, and this can sometimes lead to a variety of misunderstandings and unnecessary distress.

There are times when people choose to ignore their symptoms, perhaps because they are frightened or they do not understand their significance. This may have an important effect on the potential success of treatment outcomes. This is the case with breast cancer, where early treatment – when the cancer is still quite small and has not spread beyond the breast – appears to offer the best hope of cure (Facione 1993). Health professionals can help people to recognize potentially serious symptoms and encourage them to seek medical help. However, they may also wish to help them to recognize that minor illnesses, such as colds or flu, are best treated at home using simple remedies.

Exercise

How do people decide what causes a disease or illness? What causes a cold, influenza or breast cancer? Now ask the same members of your family you asked to define health. Are there any differences between your list and theirs? Why might that be?

Lay people usually give different reasons for illnesses than health professionals. It appears that these 'lay representations' have five components (Leventhal and Nerenz 1982; Lau and Hartman 1983). It is important for nurses and therapists to realize that patients will probably be seeking information about each of these five components:

1 *Identity* – the name of the disease.
2 *Consequences* – what will happen to me?
3 *Time line* – the duration of the illness.
4 *Causes* – why has this happened to me?
5 *Cure* – what can be done about it?

Identity is the label, or name of the disease, provided by the doctor. It is generally very worrying to be uncertain about what is wrong with you. Many patients attend hospital for investigation of their symptoms and it should be appreciated that they are likely to be very worried about the outcome of medical investigations. It is a paradox that some patients will express relief even when they are given a potentially life-threatening diagnosis like cancer, because they find prolonged uncertainty difficult to tolerate. There are some diseases like multiple sclerosis which are notoriously difficult to diagnose. There is often a long delay between the appearance of symptoms and the patient being given a definite diagnosis. During this time, the patient will be actively searching for a meaning for their strange symptoms of weakness, slurred speech or visual disturbance. It often comes as a relief for them to know that they are not lazy or mad. These issues are highlighted again in Chapter 8 in the section on chronic pain.

Once a disease has an identity, people think about the *consequences*. There is an important role here for nurses, midwives and therapists in helping people to understand what the future may hold. In some conditions, like multiple sclerosis, it is very difficult to predict the extent of residual neurological damage. It may help patients and families to talk with an occupational therapist and learn about the help that can be provided to facilitate daily living. Linked to consequences is the *time line* or expected duration of an illness. We can often be very confident in predicting that in a few days we will feel better after getting a cold. Yet in multiple sclerosis and many other chronic diseases, it is almost impossible to tell individual patients what will happen to them. We can give them estimates of probability that they will become disabled, but such information is not very helpful at an individual level.

People often want to know the *cause* of their disease. It seems that people make an active search for meaning, even if there is no medical certainty about causation. It is known that breast cancer patients often ask the question 'why me?' It may be helpful for people to make attributions about causation, as it provides a sense of being in control of one's life and creates less of a feeling that arbitrary events can change the world. Perceptions of personal control and a rejection of fate may be a Western phenomenon. In a study of British people's beliefs about their current and future health, most people strongly rejected the role of chance, fate or supernatural powers (like God) in influencing their health (Furnham 1994).

FOCUS ON

RESEARCH

Cultural factors in the perception of disease

Baider and De-Nour (1986) studied 10 Muslim Arab women living in Israel. All the women had breast cancer and had been treated by mastectomy. The researchers interviewed the women to find out about their attributions about the cause of breast cancer. It is important to know a little bit about Arab Islamic culture to understand their responses. Islam has a belief system which places a high value on religion, tradition, the family unit and sexual modesty. An important aspect of the belief system is the concept of destiny. These are some of the attributions made by the women (p. 9):

> God gives us our bodies and God takes our bodies. There is nothing more that can be said.

> Fate is written in the Book like the day one is born and the day one dies.

> It is not in our power to decide our destiny. You, or doctors, cannot help me because it is beyond human decisions. Illnesses are part of our destiny.

> It is God's will what happens to me, and I am here just to obey God. God is with me and my fate is his.

Finally, people make judgements about how diseases are *cured*, or how people recover from them. Health professionals can provide information about treatments. Many people are quite gloomy and underestimate the cure rate of cancer, for example. Once again, chronic diseases represent a special case, as people cannot be cured but the condition may be controlled. Lau and Hartman (1983) suggested that attributions concerning getting sick and getting better may be conceptualized along three dimensions: stability, locus and controllability. *Stability* refers to the relative consistency of symptoms over time; *locus* relates to attributions that are made about the perceived source of the problem, whether internal (my own fault) or external (due to others, or the situation); and *controllability* refers to perception of an individual's ability to control the disease or cause. Imagine that a person has a cold. They are likely to think that the runny nose and sore throat, although unpleasant, will be gone in a few days (stability dimension). They may think that the cold results from the evening they spend with friends who were all sneezing and coughing (locus dimension) and they might believe that there is probably not much they can do to get rid of the cold (controllability dimension). These concepts are developed in Chapters 4, 6 and 9.

It is important to remember that when we are dealing with patients, we must not assume that they will necessarily share our ideas about disease causation. Equally, we should not judge alternative understandings of illness as wrong because they are not within a Western biomedical framework. It is helpful, as part of a holistic assessment, to elicit patients' explanations of their illness. Their explanations should be accepted and not ridiculed, although you may want to offer the patient alternative explanations based on the medical understanding of their disease.

Social cognition models of health behaviour

People receive a great deal of advice from health professionals, but they do not always heed it. Do you smoke? Eat junk food? Exercise regularly? We often know what behaviours are needed to prevent disease and live a healthy life but we do not always comply with this advice. It is of interest to know what influences these decisions in order to improve the cost-effectiveness of health promotion and education. The first part of this chapter has provided an important background, from anthropology and sociology, about people's explanations of health and illness. The second part will examine psychological models that have attempted to predict how people make choices about their lifestyles and change their behaviour to influence their health. Two influential social cognition theories are outlined and discussed. These are termed 'social cognition' (or sometimes 'sociocognitive') theories because they are concerned with how people think about issues and reach decisions within a social context.

Health psychologists are particularly interested in the role of beliefs and intentions in determining health-related behaviours. Both models outlined below are based upon the assumption that people base their behaviour upon rational, conscious choices.

Health belief model

The most popular model is the health belief model (HBM; Becker and Rosenstock 1984). This model was first developed by Hochbaum in the 1950s in order to understand why so many people failed to attend for chest X-ray screening for tuberculosis (TB) (Rosenstock 1974a), and has since undergone a number of modifications.

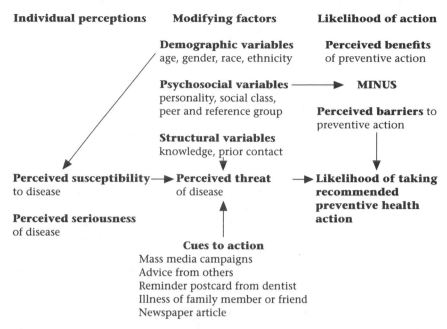

Figure 2.1 The health belief model (adapted from Becker and Rosenstock 1984).

As shown in Fig. 2.1, the HBM proposes that an individual's likelihood of taking health-enhancing action, like quitting smoking, taking more exercise or going for a screening test, is determined by a number of variables. The individual's perceptions are based on both the person's *perceived susceptibility* to a particular disease and by their perceptions of the probable *severity* of the physical and social consequences of getting the disease. These are influenced by three modifying factors: demographic characteristics, like age, gender, race and ethnicity; psychosocial variables, such as personality, social class, peer and reference group; and structural variables, including knowledge and prior contact with the disease. These factors combine in influencing a person's perception of the threat associated with a disease. In addition, people need cues to action, such as health promotion advice, mass media campaigns, a newspaper article, a reminder postcard from the dentist, or illness in a family member or friend. However, the actual likelihood of a person taking action to improve their health (i.e. changing their behaviour) depends on the *perceived benefits* of preventive action minus the *perceived barriers* or costs to that action. The way in which these components combine to effect action is illustrated in the case of Carol below.

Case study: Carol

Carol is a 52-year-old secretary working for a legal company. She has received in the post this morning an invitation to attend for mammography screening for breast cancer. What factors might contribute to her attending and what might prevent her from doing so?

Perceived threat

Perceived susceptibility – does she believe that she is *personally* likely to get breast cancer? She might regard breast cancer as serious but unlikely to happen to her, however if she is a member of a family in which many generations of women have developed the disease, she could think of it as very likely.
Perceived seriousness – how serious does she think the consequences of the disease would be if she had it? Carol might think that breast cancer is less serious if she associates it with lumpectomy, rather than mastectomy.

Demographic variables – what difference might Carol's age (e.g. 24, 48 or 74 years) make to her perceptions of threat?
Psychosocial variables – who is Carol's reference group? What difference might this make to her perceptions of threat or likelihood of taking action?
Structural variables – does Carol know about the reasons for screening?
Cues to action – if Carol's aunt has recently died of breast cancer, this might mean she is more likely to attend.

Cost–benefit analysis

Perceived benefits – she may believe that she will be reassured that she does not have the disease or, if she does have it, confident that it can be treated successfully at an early stage.
Perceived barriers – these may include inconvenience of the appointment time or place, embarrassment, belief that mammography is painful, or fear of finding something wrong.

So what is the likelihood of Carol going for mammography? Evidence suggests (Rosenstock 1974b) that the most important variables are perceived susceptibility (people are unlikely to take action if they do not feel personally at risk) and perceived benefits versus barriers. Fear of finding something wrong can act as a huge deterrent to taking screening action, although this component has been omitted from some questionnaires based upon the HBM. For example, Champion (1984) omitted fear of finding a lump from her instrument designed to test the HBM in relation to breast self-examination.

The HBM was originally designed to understand behaviours which were related to secondary prevention, such as attending for screening and compliance with medical treatments. This explains the disease focus of the model. It has since been applied within primary prevention to try to explain a variety of health-related behaviours. One of the important problems with this is that most behaviours which influence health, such as smoking, eating, drinking, exercise and sexual activity, are not primarily influenced by health consequences. We engage in them because we gain pleasure from them, not because they are good for us, and we may be reluctant to change them because someone now tells us they are bad for us. Therefore, the HBM may be less relevant in explaining these types of behaviour and behaviour change. In addition, evidence suggests that people have fairly vague ideas about what is good or bad for them to do. In a study of women's beliefs about breast cancer causation and treatment (Payne 1990), people regarded dietary changes and stress reduction, as well as orthodox medical treatment, as important. Therefore, the actions they take may not be those which the health professionals think are most desirable.

> **Exercise**
>
> Try to apply the health belief model to a health-related behaviour that you are intending to undertake or change in the near future. Suggestions include: a check-up at the dentist, starting an exercise class/new sport, drinking less alcohol. Work through the HBM carefully and write down each part. Then monitor your behaviour. Did your behaviour match your analysis? If not, why not?

Theory of planned behaviour

The theory of planned behaviour (TPB; Ajzen 1991), like the HBM, has evolved over the last 20 years. Unlike the HBM, the TPB is designed to explain *any* behaviour, such as buying a car or choosing a shirt. Originally the 'theory of reasoned action' (TRA; Ajzen and Fisbein 1980), included just two variables personal *attitude* towards the behaviour and the *subjective norm* (what other important people would think I should do) – which were directly related to the intention to act. This was later extended (see Fig. 2.2) to include the component of *perceived personal control* (I could do it if I wanted to).

The TPB is based on the assumption that behaviours are under volitional control. As shown in Fig. 2.2, an intention to perform a behaviour is proposed as being the immediate determinant of action. The *intention* is determined by three factors. The first is the *attitude towards the behaviour*, which is simply a value judgement about whether the behaviour is a good thing or not. These attitudes are based on beliefs about the outcome of the action and an evaluation of that outcome. The second factor is the influence that a *subjective norm* or *social norm* has over the person. This refers to the subjective beliefs about the expectations of significant others regarding the action, combined with the motivation of the individual to comply with those expectations. The third factor is an assessment of the amount of *personal control* people perceive themselves to have over the particular action. This is closely related to the concepts of self-efficacy and locus of control, which are considered further in Chapters 4 and 6. It is based on an appraisal of the internal influences on taking action (including having the necessary skills and abilities) versus external factors (such as opportunities, reliance on others and economic constraints).

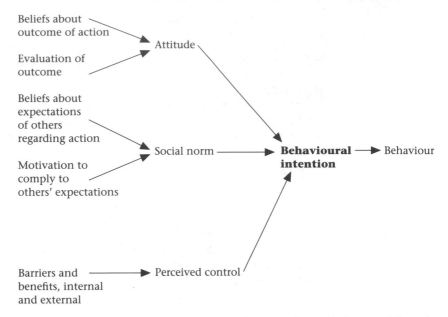

Figure 2.2 The theory of reasoned action/theory of planned behaviour (adapted from Ajzen 1991).

Case study: Barbara

Suppose you have just spent the last 15 minutes giving advice to Barbara, a 32-year-old mother, about her 20 cigarettes-a-day smoking habit. You have discussed the undesirable effects which passive smoking is likely to have on her two children (such as increased probability of respiratory conditions) and her partner's health. You have mentioned the long-term consequences for her own health and then provided her with advice and leaflets about giving up smoking. She seems convinced by your arguments and says she really wants to give up this time.

Using the TPB, Barbara's intention to quit smoking is influenced by:

- *Attitude* – Barbara's attitude that quitting smoking would be a good thing to do is determined (1) by her beliefs about the outcome ('I will be healthier and save money') and (2) her evaluation of the outcome ('Having more money to spend on the children will be worthwhile').
- *Subjective or social norm* – Barbara's attitude is that most people do not approve of smoking now. Her attitude is influenced (1) by her belief that 'My family and friends don't approve of my smoking' and (2) her motivation to comply with their wishes ('I want to quit for their sake').

- *Perceived control* – Barbara's perception of her ability to quit smoking is determined by the ratio of inhibitory and facilitatory factors that are personal to her; for example (1) 'I have the necessary information on how to quit' and (2) 'This is a good time to quit as my partner has just stopped smoking'. Therefore, 'I can do it if I want to'.

Exercise

How confident are you that Barbara will actually give up smoking? Now list all the reasons why Barbara's intentions may or may not translate into action. Which are likely to be the strongest reasons? Discuss these with your friends – what do they think? What are the implications for health education?

Advantages and disadvantages of the social cognitive models

The HBM and the TPB provide reasonable explanations for how people make choices about behaviours which are health-related. They both assume that people make logical cost–benefit analyses upon which they base their behaviour. The advantage of such models for psychologists and health care professionals is that they enable them to think carefully about each of the factors that may be involved in promoting healthy behaviours. The problem is that, although it is an advantage to have a theoretical model to guide research in this area, these models have not been found to predict behaviour very accurately. Changing people's behaviour is actually much more complicated than merely giving advice and handing out health information leaflets.

There are a number of reasons why these models are not very good at predicting behaviour. The most important is the assumption that behaviours are based upon a process of reasoning. In reality, most people do not think long and hard about everyday behaviours like brushing their teeth. These types of behaviour become automatic or **habitual**. Unfortunately, as well as good habitual behaviours like teeth brushing, we can also acquire bad habits like smoking or snacking on chocolate. Often, these behaviours become so automatic that it is hard to recognize that we are doing them. Overweight people often claim, quite correctly, that they only ever eat small meals, but they often neglect to mention the three bars of chocolate they consume each evening without even noticing. Hunt and Martin (1988) provide a good analysis of these issues and suggest that daily life needs some kind of interruption which brings a habit into focus, so that it can be changed. An example would be meeting a new partner who does not smoke, or who is keen on exercise. They also suggest that new behaviours are unlikely to be maintained until they have become habits and take place without having to think about them.

Another problem with social cognition models is that they fail to take account of the immediacy of the outcomes. The pleasurable effects of smoking or having unprotected sexual intercourse are both immediate and certain, while the health (disease) consequences are uncertain and probably a long time hence (unless disease symptoms are already apparent). Walker (1993) has argued that, for these reasons, merely giving information that something may damage your health is unlikely to lead to a change in these types of behaviour. The factors which influence behaviour directly are presented in Chapter 4, where an example of a smoking prevention programme, based upon some of them, is given.

Another important problem is that many health-related behaviours are actually coping strategies which people use for dealing with stress. Smoking, drinking, eating and sex are all examples of behaviours which many people use to help cope with stressful situations. Therefore, the best of intentions may come to nothing if the individual is exposed to stressful circumstances, unless alternative strategies are available to them. This is why stress management is an important component of empowering people to change.

Research with the TPB indicates that the model is reasonably good at predicting intentions (Ajzen 1988), but poor at predicting actual behaviour (e.g. Calnan and Rutter 1986, 1988). For example, a person may genuinely intend to attend a screening clinic, but there may be good reasons why they never get there. For example, they may have no transport or be unable to get time off work or the children are ill. In fact, the longer the gap between expressing intentions and taking action, the less likely the action will take place (this is discussed further in Chapter 9). Therefore, an immediate demonstration of commitment is desirable.

Perhaps the most serious criticism of the HBM and the TPB is their emphasis on individual behaviour, rather than on social context. Ingham (1993) has argued that most human behaviour occurs in social situations which impose implicit and explicit constraints on the range of responses which are available to individuals. He pointed out that we practise, or fail to practise, appropriate health behaviours not through ignorance but because of the social situation we find ourselves in. Ingham has studied young people's sexual behaviour in the light of concerns about the spread of HIV/AIDS, and recommendations for people to practise 'safe sex'. He found that most first sexual experiences were unplanned and therefore protection was not used. Many young people felt that it was unnecessary to use a condom if their partner came from a good background, since they 'weren't like that'. He also pointed out that it is very difficult for a young teenage girl to ask an older boy, to whom she is attracted and is afraid of losing, to use a condom. Not only do young adolescent girls lack the skills of social negotiation, but they may feel relatively powerless to do so. For this reason, Ingham has recommended assertiveness training as an important component of life-skills education for girls.

Ingham pointed out that data collected in research using social cognition models are usually based on questionnaires. Yet there is much confusion about the use of words when not everyone has access to the same vocabularies. Certain words used to describe sexual function or organs are only used in certain situations – for instance, as a joke, or to insult another person, or to express feelings with your partner. You may find it inappropriate to use these to talk with a patient. Evidence from research using discourse analysis (the detailed study of the way people use language to understand and construct their worlds) identifies a number of different ways of talking (and by implication thinking) about heterosexual behaviour. For instance, the *male sexual drive* discourse, the *have-hold* discourse and the *permissive* discourse (Hollway 1984). Each of these represent ways of talking about sexual behaviour. For example, sayings like young men need 'to sow their wild oats' are indicative of the male sexual drive discourse. Interestingly, there may be very different sexual behaviour discourses for men and women. Do you think this is reflected in the acceptance of different sexual behaviours for men and women in our society?

The answers that many people give to questions on questionnaires about how they would behave fall into the 'it all depends on the situation' category. When we are in social situations, we are influenced by the people around us. For instance, when we are with a group of friends, we have a reputation and a social identity to maintain. On a trip to the pub, we may not want to appear like a wimp, because we cannot keep up with the other people's alcohol consumption or choose to switch to soft drinks. There are also social norms about turn-taking in buying rounds of drinks which a person might violate if they stopped drinking or even cut down on the quantity consumed. Our behaviour may be different depending upon whether we are in the pub with our family, friends or acquaintances.

Finally, the questionnaires which are used to test these models are rarely available for inspection by the reader. However, the results depend upon the validity and reliability of the questionnaire. The authors normally report that these have been tested, but readers do not have the opportunity to judge for themselves. Weak predictions may be due not to flaws in the models themselves, but to poor validity in the construction of the instruments used to test them.

Overall, it seems that there are limits to rational behaviour, and therefore limits to the use of cognitively based models. It is therefore unwise to assume that presenting health education information to people will enable them to change their behaviour. You are invited to reconsider these issues as you read further into this book.

Exercise

Think about a recent occasion when you performed a behaviour which might potentially damage your health (e.g. driving too fast, eating chocolate bars, having 'too many' alcoholic drinks). Now write a detailed account of what happened – pretend you are an outside observer. When did the behaviour occur? What was the situation? Who else was present? Use your answers to identify what were the most important influences on your behaviour at the time.

Providing health-related advice

Health professionals often provide health promotion advice in the course of everyday interactions with clients. In fact, nurses have been urged to regard this as an important part of their role. An important area of health counselling is to do with sexual behaviour, particularly for people who seek testing for HIV. Silverman *et al.* (1992) studied HIV/AIDS counselling sessions at ten medical centres in Britain, the USA and Trinidad. They were interested in how advice was given and how it was received. They audiotaped actual sessions. Overall, they found that counsellors were more successful if they provided personalized advice, after their client had voiced his or her concerns, rather than generalized advice which could be applied to anyone. The researchers were able to identify that personalized advice elicited what they called 'marked acknowledgement' from the client, which were comments on the advice offered or further questions. In comparison, generalized advice was responded to with 'unmarked acknowledgements', which were comments like 'yes', 'mmm', 'right'. However, they found that many episodes in the counselling sessions were of generalized rather than personalized advice-giving. Why should this be?

Silverman and his colleagues suggested that there are a number of reasons which make generalized advice-giving functional for the counsellor and organization, even if it does not address the needs of the client. First, they noted that it takes much longer to elicit from clients what they see as problems or concerns. In organizational terms, appointment times needed to be longer and more resources were needed to offer a personalized service. Second, by offering generalized advice, the counsellors could avoid many potentially embarrassing difficulties of talking about an actual person's sexual behaviour. It is often much easier to talk about sexual behaviour in general, than to ask someone what they actually do. This reduces the level of potential embarrassment for both counsellor and client. By focusing on informational advice which is given to 'everyone', the counsellor is shielded from appearing to comment on the personal practices of the client. Moreover, this type of advice-giving appears to be uncontentious and can be speedily delivered with little comment – either agreement or disagreement – from the client. In fact, it provides the client with an opportunity to disregard advice which appears not to be addressed to him or her without challenging the counsellor (these issues are addressed again in Chapter 9). This research demonstrates how even skilled counsellors in a specialist service may find it difficult to deliver health promotion which is relevant and usable by a client, and which potentially influences subsequent behaviours.

Exercise

This involves an observational study of health-related advice-giving in your clinical area.

1 Select a client and health professional (ask their permission first).
2 Observe an episode of advice-giving. Use an audiotape recorder if you

> are allowed to. If not, listen very carefully to what is said and write
> down everything that you can remember immediately afterwards.
> 3 How does the health professional present the advice?
> 4 Are the client's concerns elicited first?
> 5 Is the advice presented in a personalized or generalized format?
> 6 How does the client respond to this advice?
> 7 Do you think the advice will result in a change in behaviour? Try to
> justify your answer using what you have learned from this chapter.

Summary

- Disease refers to a label used to categorize a pathological condition.

- Illness is a subjective experience.

- Anthropological, sociological and psychological approaches to health
  and illness have been reviewed.

- People make attributions about illness causation based on their world
  views.

- Illness representations include: identity, consequences, time line, causes
  and cure.

- Two social cognitive models (the health belief model and the theory of
  planned behaviour) have been presented and considered.

- Discussion of these models has highlighted the social pressures which
  influence behaviour and the limits to rationality.

Further reading

Ajzen, I. (1988) *Attitudes, Personality and Behaviour*. Milton Keynes. Open
    University Press.
Hunt, S.M. and Martin, C.J. (1988) Health-related behavioural change – a
    test of a new model. *Psychology and Health*, 2: 209–30.
Murray, M. (1990) Lay representations of illness. In P. Bennett, J. Weinman
    and P. Spurgeon (eds), *Current Developments in Health Psychology*, pp. 63–
    92. London: Harwood Academic.
Radley, A. (1994) *Making Sense of Illness*. London: Sage.
Stainton Rogers, W. (1991) *Explaining Health and Illness: An Exploration of
    Diversity*. Hemel Hempstead: Harvester Wheatsheaf. Chapters 2 and 3.
Walker, J.M. (1993) A social behavioural approach to understanding and
    promoting condom use. In J. Wilson-Barnett and J. Macleod Clark (eds),
    Research in Health Promotion and Nursing. Basingstoke: Macmillan.

SELF CONCEPT AND BODY IMAGE

Introduction

Much of the work undertaken by nurses and therapists directly involves other people's bodies. For example, helping to lift someone up in bed, measuring pulse and blood pressure, and so on. These sorts of things include touching people, sometimes in ways which are potentially very embarrassing, such as in undertaking a catheterization. How do we learn to cope with dealing with other people's bodies? How do people think and feel about their own bodies? Different societies have different strict taboos on which parts of the body can be exposed where, what can be seen and by whom. How should this influence health care provision in a multicultural society? Research by Lawler (1991) has shown how nursing work involves a detailed social understanding of the body, to which the reader may wish to refer. This is why a whole chapter in this book is devoted to these issues.

A humanistic perspective on the concept of self was introduced in Chapter 1. This chapter will focus upon two important aspects of the self concept: body image and self-esteem. It will include theoretical models of how children learn about their bodies and understand how they function in health and sickness. It will review research on patients who have head and neck cancer because they represent a special group of people who have to cope with major changes in their body image. Consideration will be given to how changes in facial appearance can affect the way other people react to them, and the impact this might have on the way people think and feel about themselves. The part that self-esteem plays in helping people to cope with everyday life and stressful events, like being ill, are discussed. Finally, the chapter will consider how knowledge about body image and self-esteem can be used in communication with people in health care settings.

Children's concepts of their bodies, health and illness

In the last chapter, it was suggested that adults have available to them a number of ways of understanding and talking about health and illness. The explanations they use are not arbitrary guesses or misconceptions, but are integrated with their understanding of their world. So how do children come to understand their bodies and learn about being healthy or sick? These issues are important in enabling health professionals to know how to talk with sick children. For instance, how would you talk to a 5-year-old about asthma? How would you explain the function of drugs delivered by inhaler?

FOCUS ON

RESEARCH

Children's ideas about the insides of their bodies

Eiser and Patterson (1983) interviewed four groups of 26 children who were aged 6, 8, 10 and 12 years. These children were all healthy and attending normal school. The children were asked to draw what was inside their body on an outline diagram. An adult helped them to label the organs. On another outline diagram they were asked to draw a circle where the following organs were located: heart, brain, stomach, lungs, kidney, liver and bladder. Finally, they were asked what parts of their body were needed for eating, breathing, getting rid of waste and swimming. Perhaps not surprisingly, the children were able to identify more body parts as they got older. On average, the 6-year-olds could identify three, the 8-year-olds four, the 10-year-olds six, and the 12-year-olds seven. When all the children's responses were grouped together, the most frequently mentioned organs were the brain (76 per cent), heart (74 per cent), bones (71 per cent), blood (58 per cent) and lungs (38 per cent), while only two children mentioned the sexual organs. All of the children knew that the mouth and stomach were involved in eating, but few of them were aware of digestive processes or that food was absorbed into the bloodstream. Some 6-year-olds did not know what organs were involved in breathing, although, with increasing age, the heart and lungs were mentioned more frequently. Twenty-one of the 6-year-olds appeared to know nothing about 'getting rid of waste' and were unable to answer the question about this, although there was an increase in knowledge with age. Finally, most of the children knew that the arms and legs were needed for swimming; however, the younger children related this to the bones, while 54 per cent of the 12-year-olds talked about the role of the brain in controlling activity.

This study is useful because it provides us with detailed information about how much children of different ages know about their bodies. It also makes clear that there is a major difference between children being able to draw the heart, use the word 'heart', and their understanding·of the function of the heart. In fact, very young children may say that the heart is 'for loving' but have no idea of its role as a pump. This is an important factor to remember when we are dealing with adults who may use words like stomach to mean a general area of the abdomen extending from below the ribs to the pubic bone. This has a rather different meaning from the medical definition of a specific J-shaped digestive organ at the base of the oesophagus. Children tend to regard health as being about doing things like running around and playing. They assign a central role to diet, but appear to understand little about digestion.

Children growing up in Britain will be taught about human biology at school, so that their improved understanding of functional processes as they grow older is probably attributable in part to the educational system. Nevertheless, viewers of Bruce Forsyth's television show may have witnessed amazingly poor scores on the placing of body organs by adults. It is also worth remembering that this is based upon an organic model and some might argue that, just as one does not need to know the workings of an internal combustion engine to drive a car, people do not need to know details of their inner bodies in order to function healthily. This is illustrated by the issues raised in Chapter 2. Health professionals need to use different levels of communication according to age, education and belief systems.

Theoretical models of children's understanding of health and illness

There has been an attempt to relate children's understanding to their level of cognitive development. Piaget, the 'father' of developmental psychology, proposed that children proceed through a number of sequential stages as they learn to make sense of their world. At each of these stages, the child thinks in qualitatively different ways. Piaget emphasized that this was different from a purely maturational approach. (It may help you to look up Piaget's developmental theory in a basic psychology textbook before reading the next section.) Based upon interviews with children of different ages, Bibace and Walsh (1981) proposed a six-stage model within a Piagetian framework to account for children's understanding of health and illness. The ages are approximate:

1 *Phenomenism* (ages 2–4). At the earliest age, children see the cause of illness as an external object which may occur at the same time as other phenomena but be remote from them. For example:

> *Adult*: How do people get colds?
> *Child*: From the sun.
> *Adult*: How does the sun give you a cold?
> *Child*: It just does that's all.

2 *Contagion* (ages 4–7). The cause of illness is seen to be in objects or people close to the child, but the link between the two is poorly understood or accounted for by supernatural processes. For example:

> *Adult*: How do people get colds?
> *Child*: When somebody comes near you.
> *Adult*: How?
> *Child*: I don't know, by magic I think.

3 *Contamination* (ages 7–9). By about 7 years of age, illnesses are seen as being caused either through touch or the child engaging in harmful actions or being 'bad'. For example:

> *Adult*: How do you get a rash?
> *Child*: If somebody has got a rash, and you touch them, you get it.

4 *Internalization* (ages 9–11). Illness is now seen to be located within the body, although the causes may be external. For example:

> *Adult*: How do you get a cold?
> *Child*: You breath in cold air and get a cough.

5 *Physiological* (ages 11–16). By about 11 or 12 years of age, explanations for illness are given in terms of malfunctioning of specific organs. Attributions of causation are likely to focus on physical factors. For example:

> *Adult*: How do people get colds?
> *Child*: There are viruses in the air which people inhale, which causes them to have a cough and runny nose.

6 *Psychophysiological* (age 16 and above, although some people never reach this stage). In the final stage, children realize that a person's thoughts and feelings can affect the way in which the body functions. For example:

> *Adult*: How do people get colds?
> *Child*: There are viruses in the air which people inhale, and if they are feeling run down or under stress they might develop a cold.

Bibace and Walsh (1981) suggest that children cannot understand an explanation of illness in advance of their cognitive development. So that when we talk to 6-year-olds about asthma, it is pointless trying to get them to understand what happens in their lungs. They suggest that children use the logic which is available to them at each Piagetian cognitive stage. For instance, children up to Piaget's operational stage (about the age of 7 years) do not realize that a spherical lump of clay can be rolled out into a long sausage without changing its weight; or water poured from a short, fat container to a tall, thin container without changing its amount or volume. They may attribute these transformations to 'magic' or similar processes.

Exercise

Using the Bibace and Walsh model, describe how you might explain diabetes to a 3-year-old, an 8-year-old and an 18-year-old. How would you explain why they needed to have insulin injections? How would you check what they have understood? Why would your explanations vary for each individual?

How useful do you think that this model is? Can you think of any problems with it? Does it fit with the experience you have had with children? Some children, especially those with chronic diseases, actually seem to have very sophisticated knowledge about their conditions. Eiser (1990) has suggested that it may be possible to account for the changes in children's understanding by looking at their everyday experiences rather than relating them to their cognitive developmental level. She points out that very young children are often not offered explanations by adults and may be provided with sayings like 'an apple a day keeps the doctor away' without an explanation of why. Older children may have some experience of contagious diseases or picking things up (e.g. nits) from other children. Teenagers are exposed to media reporting of, for example, the role of stress in heart disease, and they may be taught health studies in school. Alternative approaches have acknowledged that children have less practical experience than adults. This might account for the age-related differences they tend to show in their understanding of health and illness.

It is interesting to note the epistemological (origins of knowledge) similarities between the development of explanations about health and illness in the growing child and the evolution of social accounts of illness through history. It is not so long since bacterial diseases were generally thought to be spread by bad air. For example, post-natal infections (the major cause of maternal death after the introduction of institutionalized maternity care following the industrial revolution) were thought to be spread via this 'miasma'. Semmelweis, during the mid-nineteenth century, was not initially believed when he asserted that these infections were spread by the unwashed hands of doctors examining patient after patient.

Scripts and schemas in understanding health care

Nelson (1986) proposed a 'script' theory. She suggests that children (and adults for that matter) represent knowledge of events in abstract schemas. (Scripts and schemas are usually included under memory theory and are referred to again in Chapter 5.) **Schemas** are mental representations of the events which are associated with a particular situation. They may be based upon past experiences or external sources of information and allow individuals to make predictions about what will occur. A **script** refers to the routine pattern of behaviour which the individual expects to follow in a particular situation. For example, an out-patient clinic visit script may contain the following: when you first arrive you give the doctor's letter to the receptionist; then you are directed to the right clinic; you sit down and wait; a nurse weighs you and asks you for a specimen of urine; you wait again; you see the doctor in an office; you are asked to go into another room and undress; you are then examined; you get dressed again; the doctor tells you what s/he has found; you make another appointment; you collect your medication from the pharmacy; you go home. All of this might come as no surprise to you if you have been to an out-patient appointment. Moreover, having this information in your head allows you to predict what will happen and gives you a feeling of being in control. Schemas tell us what to expect, while scripts tell us how to behave. For example, if we go to a hospital clinic we may expect to spend some time waiting, so we might take a book or magazine to read, whereas if we go for a private consultation we would not expect to wait to see the doctor. People without a schema may feel frightened because they are unable to predict what will happen next. Being asked to produce a urine sample if you are not expecting it can come as an embarrassing shock. A schema may require modification – for example, if having a blood test or X-ray is added to a subsequent clinic visit. Nelson suggests that children lack experience of life and therefore lack explanatory schemas. She suggested that their errors are due to a lack of experience rather than a different way of thinking.

Research has demonstrated that even young children have schemas and scripts for everyday events like going to the supermarket, eating at McDonalds and baking a cake (Nelson 1986). In an unpublished study, Payne asked 5-year-old children about what happens when they go to the doctor and the dentist, and found that most of them were able to provide a detailed description of what happens in a logical sequence of activity. She asked the same children about what happens when they go to hospital or have an operation. Once again, most of the children could say what happens when you go to hospital. Unlike adult 'scripts', they tended to include a lot of details about eating and playing which, of course, are very salient for children. There were more problems in eliciting an 'operation script', and quite a few children, even some 8-year-olds, did not understand what the word meant.

Health care professionals can provide information which will allow people to develop schemas and scripts about medical procedures. For example, having blood pressure measured involves a cuff being placed around the upper arm. The cuff becomes progressively tighter as it is inflated, which might cause tingling in the fingers but there is only a short period of discomfort. This description enables the patient to predict what is likely to happen and prevents them having unpleasant surprises. It may contribute to a perception of feeling in control. It also allows people to behave in appropriate ways and avoid embarrassment. Learning can be from direct experience or gained vicariously by observing others, such as in watching television dramas. Some of the children stated that they knew about what happens in hospitals from watching 'Children's Ward'.

Exercise

Elicit a nursing or medical 'script' (a suggestion might include having blood taken) from five patients and five people who are not receiving health care. Does everyone have a 'script' for your chosen event? (Remember 'scripts' are descriptions of behaviour patterns which are sequentially ordered.) What are the common features of these scripts? How do they differ? Why do you think that might be?

Self concept

All psychologists (with the exception of behaviourists for whom the issue is considered to be irrelevant) have attempted to explore people's subjective understanding of their internal 'self'. A humanistic account of the self concept was introduced in Chapter 1. An important account of the development of the self concept has emerged from social psychology. Social psychologists have suggested that we learn about our own self through comparing ourselves with others. Leon Festinger (1954) termed this **social comparison theory**. Comparisons may be objective within a particular **reference group**, but are also relative since they depend upon who our reference group is. For example, those who are 5 feet 8 inches tall are considered tall if they are women and short if they are men; short if they are American and tall if they are Japanese. It seems that we make comparisons with people who are similar to ourselves, but it is important that we select an appropriate reference group to compare ourselves with.

According to Goffman (1971), an important part of an individual's self concept is determined by the *social roles* they play (this is developed further in Chapter 9). We all play a large number of social roles. For instance, as well as being a student, you may also be a lover, a friend, a daughter or son, a health worker, and so on. Some of these roles may be so familiar to you that you have difficulty in recognizing them as roles. In fact, we often become more aware of our roles as sons or daughters only once we return to our parents' home after a period away. Other roles, such as health worker, may be quite new and cause you to feel rather self-conscious at first. You may feel unsure how to act in your new role. However, after a period of 'socialization', roles become internalized and you take them for granted. Of course, there are social expectations about how we play our roles. For instance, it is expected that sons and daughters will show affection for their parents; that nurses will be kind, gentle and caring. Goffman suggested that any one person will have available to them a number of these social roles, although the performance of these roles will only be appropriate in specific social situations. This frequently differs depending on who we are with. For example, a physiotherapist might be kind and gentle with a worried client, but noisy or comical with friends. Thus our sense of self is somewhat determined by the social situation we are currently in. We sometimes cause offence if we misjudge the social role of another person. It may not be appreciated if we refer to an elderly gentleman as 'grandpa', since he may feel that he does not fit into that role in a hospital situation.

It is often quite difficult to make transitions between the roles we play. You may have noticed that parents have a difficult transition in adjusting their role in relation to their adolescent children. Linville (1987) found that people vary in their ability to perceive themselves differently in different situations. Some people have a unified self schema and think of themselves as having the same attributes in every situation and in every role. Others have clearly differentiated self schemas and think of themselves as having quite different attributes in different roles and situations. Having a complex self concept appears to make people more adaptive and resilient to stress-related illness and depression.

> **Exercise**
>
> Think about the roles you play. Try to identify as many roles as possible. Now think about the characteristics which make up these roles. How many are similar and how many are different? Do the demands of these roles ever conflict with each other? If so, how do you deal with these and how do they make you feel?

Sometimes, comparisons can lead to false self-appraisals. For example, people who suffer from anorexia often appear to judge themselves to be overweight when they are actually very underweight in relation to the population of their age and sex. Comparisons are commonly made with other family members, as illustrated in Chapter 1. A bright offspring may judge him or herself to be rather dim and as a consequence underachieve, if persistently compared to an older sibling who is exceptionally intelligent. In fact, families tend to make comparisons from the time a child is born and these may lay the foundations for later self-comparisons.

> **Exercise**
>
> Next time you spend time in a baby clinic, or visit a friend who has a baby or young child, record the comparisons the mother makes. On what dimensions are comparisons made? Who are the objects of the comparison? How many of the comparisons are positive and how many are negative? How do these comparisons appear to relate to the mother's feelings towards the child?

There have been a number of psychological theories based on the idea that the 'self' is central to people's understanding of the world. You may have noticed that people can have quite different views of the same event. Try discussing among your friends what their views were of a recent lecture or a visit to a pub. Some may have enjoyed it while others expressed indifference or even found it boring. The range of views may not be very great among your close friends (we tend to choose people to be our friends because they share similar views to our own), but if you ask other members of your class there may be a greater variety of responses. These views are all valid and are likely to be influenced by many factors, including motivation and past learning experiences. The phenomenological approach within humanistic psychology tries to understand each individual's unique world view, or perspective. These world views are part of our taken-for-granted way of seeing the world. Without some careful reflection, it is difficult to be aware of our own world views.

In health care, this has given rise to research which is based on describing the 'lived experience' of illness. For example, in a study of diabetic patients,

Cohen *et al.* (1994) found that patients viewed coping with the immediate lifestyle constraints of diabetes as very salient; for example, how to regulate their food and insulin requirements to accommodate unplanned tennis matches or a late night Indian meal. On the other hand, health care professionals understood diabetes in terms of preventing long-term complications, such as retinopathy and neuropathy, and they regarded the day-to-day living concerns as less salient. In fact, some people with diabetes do not regard themselves as ill (Callaghan and Williams 1994), as they have grown up with the disorder and it has become a normal part of their self concept. Research findings like these have implications for the way health professionals interact with people. It may be more appropriate for people who have chronic diseases to be partners in the management of their condition, rather than viewed as patients needing care to be provided *for* them. As people vary in their world views, it is important for carers to elicit these views when they first become involved.

Humanistic psychology emphasizes the importance of congruence between the actual self and ideal self. Kelly (1955) proposed that people's views of reality are important in guiding their behaviour. Moreover, views change in the light of everyday experiences and may be shaped by each of these episodes of learning. The example of Ann was given in Chapter 1 to illustrate how the repertory grid technique can be used to explain anxiety and low self-esteem in terms of the distance between the actual self and the ideal self. This technique has been used in a variety of therapeutic settings. A person with anorexia nervosa might have constructs such as 'thin is beautiful', 'being beautiful is good' as well as many others. Before treatment, there is often a large discrepancy in how they view their ideal self (thin, beautiful) and how they view their present self (fat, ugly). One of the ways to measure the success of therapy is to identify if there is an increase in agreement between an individual's ideal self and their present or actual self. According to Kelly's theory, anorexic people behave in relation to their perceived reality (fat, ugly), rather than using objective measures like weighing scales or mirrors.

Body image

As well as forming schemas about events in our lives and about attributes such as personality and intelligence, we also form schemas about our bodies. Body image is an important aspect of self concept for health professionals because we work with many people who are experiencing changes to their actual body. Some of these are abrupt changes resulting from trauma or surgery. Others are insidious changes resulting from disease processes like rheumatoid arthritis.

Body image is a fundamental aspect of a person's individual identity, the mental representation of who we are. According to social identity theory (Brewer 1991), one's identity results from a balance between a need to be similar to one's reference group and the need to be a unique individual. It seems we may actually have more than one identity – for example, a personal identity and a group identity. When you are at work, a uniform may provide you with a feeling of group cohesion with other nurses, midwives or therapists which can be supportive. However, when you are off duty, you probably take care not to wear exactly the same clothes as your friends. If you went to a party and found another person in the same outfit you might be very upset.

According to Price (1990), normal *body image* has three parts: reality, presentation and ideal. *Body reality* refers to the structure of individual bodies; that is, whether a person is tall, short or slim. The structure of bodies changes over time, from infancy and childhood through sexual differentiation at puberty, through middle age (and the menopause for women), to old age. At different periods in our lives, we appear to inhabit very different bodies, although, paradoxically, most people have a sense of continuity about their own bodies. Body reality can also be changed deliberately, such as going on a slimming diet or starting a weight-training programme. It may also be changed as a result of accidents or disease. Basic aspects of our body reality are determined by genetic factors like our eye and hair colour.

Exercise

Get out your family photograph album. Look at pictures of yourself as a baby, a toddler, a schoolchild and a recent one. Look at your body. Are you the same person in all the photographs? Do you feel the same?

Body presentation is about the characteristic ways in which the body moves or functions in social situations. As you probably know, gestures and physical actions, even very subtle facial movements or hand gestures, convey information to people. This is non-verbal communication. Some responses are shared by all people like raising the eyebrows as a greeting signal, while other responses are specific to cultural groups. We acquire these behaviours and use them in a largely unconscious way. In fact, we may feel very awkward if we try to suppress these behaviours, such as keeping our hands still when talking. When these responses are changed by a disease process, it can make interactions appear very difficult and uncomfortable, such as with a person who has Parkinson's disease and whose face shows very little movement.

Exercise

Next time you are working in a clinical area, note the body presentation of the other staff. How do people use their hands? Look at their body posture. Is it upright or inclined towards the patient? Does it vary with the status or grade of the health professional? Try not to make it obvious that you are watching as people will then become very self-conscious and change their behaviours.

Finally, people have a concept of their *ideal body* (part of their ideal sense of self). This is likely to be gender- and age-specific. It is also likely to be influenced by cultural norms which define appropriate size, shape and contours. In Britain, women's magazines provide information not only about current fashions, but on appropriate body shape and colour, for example urging women to be slim and suntanned. Recent concerns about the role of sunburn in the causation of skin cancer has led to media advice about 'safe' tanning and the use of sun-screening creams. A brief look at a history of fashion book will show how women's – and to a lesser extent men's – ideal body shapes have varied over the decades. There are also cultural norms about the body space, that area around the person which is regarded as private. Health care professionals need to be sensitive to people's feelings of vulnerability when this space is invaded. Formation of a personal body ideal involves a process of comparison between perceptions of one's real body, cultural norms, and perceptions of one's reference group. If the ideal body image shows a major discrepancy from the perceived reality of the body, the person may feel very dissatisfied with their body. This might lead them to take action such as seeking cosmetic surgery. As noted in Chapter 1, reality is a contentious issue. It is probably better to think of body image being based on people's perceptions. This might account for why some very obese people believe themselves to be of 'normal' weight and people with anorexia nervosa starve themselves to death. These people may be regarded as having a distorted body image.

We not only have an image of our own bodies but also hold an image of members of our close family and friends. One of the distressing aspects of caring for a person with advanced cancer is the changes brought about by cachexia. The wasting of the person's body can be so severe that relatives fail to recognize their loved one as the same person they shared their life with.

Stigma

It has already been suggested that body image is not just dependent upon our own evaluations of ourselves, but is heavily influenced by the responses of others to us. Goffman (1968b), a sociologist, first introduced the concept of stigma. A stigma refers to an outward sign which damages the self concept of the person. Goffman described three types of stigma:

1 Moral stigma – behaviour or attributes which violate cultural or social values.
2 Tribal stigma – features or adornments which signal group membership.
3 Physical stigma – deviations from normal appearance which may be interpreted as deformity or disfigurement.

Moral stigma refers to attributes of the individual which are regarded as morally reprehensible in a particular culture. For example, it is accepted in most cultures that killing another human being is unlawful, although the punishment and resulting stigma is tempered by the circumstances of the killing. Causing death by reckless driving (under the influence of alcohol) is generally punished less severely than killing a person while engaged in a robbery. Recently, pressure groups in North America and Britain have campaigned for this offence to be taken more seriously. There appears to be increasing public intolerance of drunk driving, which is now a stigmatized activity. Moral stigma may be acquired by an activity or be inherited. For example, an illegitimate birth was in the past regarded as stigmatizing, but not any longer.

Tribal stigma refers to signs which mark out a racial or ethnic group member, for example the wearing of special clothing or jewellery. Human beings commonly display their status by body adornment. In Britain, married women – and some married men – wear gold rings on the third finger of their left hand. This is a public symbol of their status. In parts of India, women use a red dot on the forehead to mark their marital status. Try to find out what other cultural groups use to signify married relationship status. Symbols as such are not stigmatizing, but they do mean that certain groups can be identified and may become the object of discrimination. In health care we need to be aware that some people may wish to continue wearing their symbols in hospital. We would not normally expect British married women to remove their wedding rings before surgery.

Physical stigma refers to alterations in the body or in bodily functions that mark people out from the rest. These may be immediately identifiable things like an amputated leg, or a scarred face, or more readily concealed changes in function, like a colostomy. Some conditions like epilepsy or HIV are not readily apparent to an outside observer. People with these types of conditions have difficult choices to make about whether they self-disclose, when and to whom. If they disclose their condition, they risk being avoided; if they do not, they may fear people finding out inadvertently, for example if they have a fit. A physical stigma is an identity acquired from the reactions of other people. Children born with a disability such as blindness may be unaware of how they differ from other children when they are very young. Moreover, there is a tendency for people to generalize a particular defect into a global disability. So blind people may be treated as though they were deaf or had learning difficulties (the 'does he take sugar' syndrome).

According to Goffman, stigmatized people have to negotiate a new identity. They may use a number of tactics to do this. One alternative is to mix only with other people who share similar attributes. For example, some deaf people who use sign language may feel more comfortable in social situations where signing is the dominant communication system. They do not need to explain to others that they are deaf, nor are they stared at and made to feel abnormal when they are signing. It is often difficult for parents of deaf children to know how much to encourage their children to form relationships with other deaf people or how much they should be helped to integrate into the hearing world. Other ways of dealing with physical stigma include preparing explanations which are shared with everyone, or ignoring the disability and hoping that everyone else does as well.

To have a normal body that is pain free and functional is a central part of most people's self concept. However, facial appearance is also of great importance to the development of a positive body image, since physical attractiveness is known to be an important component in social interaction. Parents may be very distressed by the appearance of a baby with a harelip and/or cleft palate and find it difficult to develop a close relationship. Seeing another baby who has been successfully treated can be very reassuring to such parents at an early stage.

Bull (1988) has described how even a minor facial disfigurement, such as a port wine stain, can have a quite dramatic influence over the way that other people behave towards the 'stigmatized' individual. One of his studies involved marking the face of a normal individual with a port wine type stain and observing the behaviour of other passengers in a railway carriage. When the person sat with the blemish visible from the adjacent seat, other people tended to avoid sitting there until the other seats were occupied. Some of these social issues of stigmatization are considered in Chapter 9. It appears that people with physical differences, whether congenital, or acquired through injury or surgery, are probably quite right in fearing that other people will react differently towards them.

SPECIAL

TOPIC

Head and neck cancer

In this section, detailed consideration is given to a particular group of patients who have head and neck cancer. It could equally have been concerned with conditions such as severe burns, skin diseases or facial birth marks like port wine stains, that are immediately apparent to the observer. Head and neck cancers are in fact comparatively rare, accounting for just 5 per cent of all tumours. They are rather more common in men over 60 years of age who have smoked and regularly drunk alcohol. The actual cancers may occur in many sites, including the tongue, lips, mouth and larynx. Each cancer gives rise to rather different problems or defects, depending on the nature of the treatment (radiotherapy, surgery or chemotherapy) and the extent of the tumour. Extensive surgery to the face can result in major mutilation, when the soft tissues of the face and the underlying bones are removed. Patients may be provided with a prosthesis (artificial replacement), which may replace a missing eye or part of the face. Although these are skilfully made, they cannot compensate for the missing live tissue. Treatment for facial cancer is difficult to disguise, especially if it results in functional changes such as loss of speech (from laryngectomy), eating or breathing difficulties. In addition, there are less well-recognized losses which may include the ability to display emotions (such as smiling and laughing) and the role of the face and mouth in intimacy and sexual contact.

Facial mutilation is a physical stigma which may involve loss of self-image and identity, since the face is the most recognizable part of most people. Changes to dentition (losing teeth) are characteristically associated with ageing. Thus surgery may be perceived to precipitate premature ageing. Actual perceptions of mutilation are based on the significance people attach to their physical appearance. It may be guessed that it is potentially more damaging for women, given social norms of the value of female beauty. Based on interviews, MacGregor (1970) found that these patients reacted with feelings of shame and fear. Some responded by avoiding all social contacts and were very isolated but protected themselves from the disgusted responses of others. Drettner and Ahlbom (1983) used a questionnaire to assess 52 patients with head and neck cancers and their responses were compared with age- and gender-matched controls. They found that patients were very anxious pre-operatively about the extent of mutilation. Although they had been prepared by the medical staff, they could only appreciate the full impact once surgery had been completed. In the long term, despite the mutilation, patients regarded themselves as healthy, and those with a good prognosis were significantly more likely to appreciate hobbies than healthy people. This perhaps indicates that quality of life is not always worse in cancer patients compared with healthy people, as the threat to life may mean that they reappraise aspects of their life. Studies have shown that patients vary in their acceptance of prostheses. Some people found them to be too conspicuous. It seems that they are beneficial in producing acceptable responses from other people, rather than in helping the person who has the disfigurement. When major changes to body image occur, it has been suggested that people experience a loss which requires a period of adaptation. The process of adaptation may have similarities to the grief response which occurs after bereavement (see Chapter 7). Patients with head and neck cancer not only have to become accustomed to their new appearance, but they have to learn to tolerate new responses from other people towards them (Koster and Bergsma 1990). Some of these social psychological issues are addressed again in Chapter 9.

From a cognitive psychological perspective, Cohen and Lazarus (1979) have identified six sources of threat posed by cancer:

- to life
- to the unmarred body
- to the self concept
- to the emotional balance
- to the fulfilment of customary social roles and activities
- from the medical setting

Exercise

Identify someone (a patient, colleague or friend) who has experienced a change in their body image. Ask them how they feel about the change. What does it mean to them? Try to find out how they have coped with the change.

Self-esteem

Self-esteem has already emerged as an important concept in humanistic and cognitive psychology. Self-esteem reflects a critical evaluative judgement of self-worth. Once again, this is based on a combination of how we perceive others to see us, together with our own appraisal of their judgements. Self-esteem has a major role to play in the psychological well-being of people. Indeed, it is part of our sense of psychological well-being.

There has been some debate among psychologists about whether self-esteem is a global attitude about one's self or a multidimensional concept. In the past, research psychologists have attempted to measure self-esteem by posing a series of scaled questions on a questionnaire and summing up the responses to produce a total score (see the Rosenberg Self Esteem Scale 1965). The following are the sort of questions used to measure self-esteem: 'All in all, I am inclined to feel that I am a failure'; 'I feel that I have a number of good qualities'.

An alternative is to consider feelings of self-worth in relation to the roles that are important to an individual. Each of these roles may be influenced by disease and treatment in different ways. For example, a mastectomy scar may affect self-esteem as a wife and/or lover, but may not impinge at all on life as a businesswoman. Of course, people's roles change throughout their lives and this raises questions about whether self-esteem is stable throughout life or whether it changes. It seems likely that there are stable elements to self-esteem which are formed early in life. However, life events, such as developing a degenerative disease or becoming unemployed, may cause people to re-evaluate aspects of themselves and lose their self-esteem.

Figure 3.1 illustrates the ways in which sense of self can be influenced by a serious accident. The case example given below elaborates on this process.

Case study: Colin

Colin is a successful 42-year-old computer software analyst. He is happily married with three teenage children who are all doing well at school. He is a keen runner, goes jogging every day and competes in local road races. One day when driving home from work, his car is hit by a lorry. He sustains severe crush injuries to his spinal cord, which result in permanent paralysis of both legs and incontinence. As you can see from Fig. 3.1, before his accident, Colin's self concept was composed of being a parent, a sexual partner, a runner and a worker. In the immediate period in hospital after his accident, all aspects of his self concept are threatened, so it may be very difficult for him to feel good about himself. During the rehabilitation phase, he realizes that he can still show interest in his children and function as a caring father. He can operate a computer. This means that in the long term he may be able to return to full-time employment. He will never be able to run again, but he may be able to compete in wheelchair races which may maintain his concept of being a sportsman.

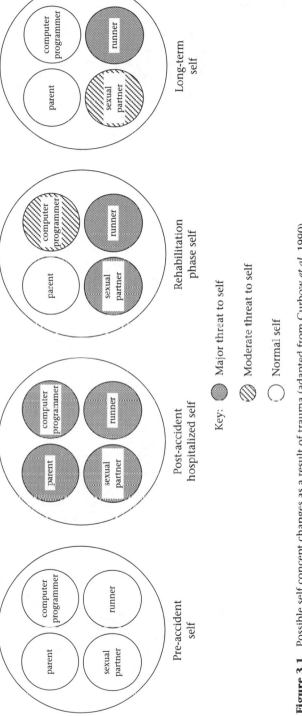

Figure 3.1 Possible self concept changes as a result of trauma (adapted from Curbow *et al.* 1990).

> **Exercise**
>
> How would you evaluate Colin's self-esteem prior to the accident and why? Record each of Colin's roles and consider the effect that changes to each are likely to have on his self-esteem. Which do you think is likely to result in the greatest damage to his self-esteem and why? Is it the role of the health care professional to assist Colin and his wife to cope with changes in their marital relationship? If so, who, when and how?

You will probably not be able to answer all of the above questions. However, they are issues which need to be addressed and resolved. Sexual difficulties, along with death and dying, are the most difficult problems which health professionals have to confront. It is tempting to think that someone else will deal with it, but they frequently do not and individuals are often left to cope alone. There are specialist psychosexual clinics where people can be helped. Self-esteem and **social support** have been closely linked in research. It is important, when confronted by an event which requires major adjustment, such as that which Colin and his wife are faced with, to know that there are people to turn to who will care and support you. In the case of injury or disease, the health care professional is an important source of knowledgeable support who can provide hope and practical advice in an atmosphere of care and understanding.

Interactions between the 'self' and the social environment

People are not passive recipients of information and social pressure from other people. It seems that people actively (although not necessarily consciously) construct their self-esteem. Curbow *et al.* (1990: 122) suggest that there are biases in the processing of self-related information. According to these researchers, 'people are inclined to focus judgement and memory on the self, perceive the self as effective in achieving desired ends, and resist cognitive changes'. This means that at times of stress, it may be difficult for people to take in information that is discrepant with their self concept. This may make it hard for them to make rational treatment decisions. It may also make people misinterpret the actions of others. In an attempt to protect their self-esteem, they may disregard health care advice, for example.

Self esteem and **social support** have been closely linked in research. We will be discussing the role of social support in helping people to cope with illness in Chapter 6. Generally, it has been found that cancer patients who have social support are more likely to have high self-esteem. This could mean that having people who love and care for you contributes to feeling good about yourself. It may also mean that people who do not feel good about themselves are unable to elicit social support from others. For example, if a person seems very unsure of themselves in social situations, they are more likely to avoid going to clubs or pubs, and thus are more likely to be relatively isolated.

In addition to our self-esteem, the evaluative element of our self concept, Bem (1967) suggests that we observe ourselves and draw conclusions about our own behaviour. You may have heard people make comments like 'I really surprised myself, I never thought I could do it' after they had achieved something like passing their driving test, or walking for the first time after an injury. Self perception is a mental representation of what we are capable of. For example, a person might perceive themselves to be timid, the sort of person who never goes on a roller-coaster. Sometimes this constrains our behaviour, so we might be too afraid to try something new. Health care professionals may have to work hard at helping people to achieve new activities like taking up a new sport. Camps for children with diabetes function in this way by allowing the children to try new experiences like canoeing or climbing which are incompatible with the perception of being an invalid. Of course, people need to succeed at the activity, if they are to change their self perception.

This chapter has reviewed evidence about the self concept; self image and self-esteem. We have seen how individuals have thoughts and feelings about themselves which are very influential in determining how they react to other people and towards themselves. Concepts of self are not immediately apparent to an observer and nurses do not routinely measure self-esteem like taking someone's temperature. Although it might be helpful to remember that just as everyone has a body temperature which fluctuates around a normal level (37C), so people also have self concepts which might also fluctuate a little depending what is happening to them and how they feel about these changes, and what the changes will mean to them in the context of their lives. When we talk to patients it is helpful to start by eliciting their understandings about how their disease or surgery might affect their body. For example, nurses are very familiar with what surgical scars look like, and they also know that scars fade with time. Patients are much less likely to have seen a scar before, and certainly not a new one. Likewise, even adults often have little understanding about their internal anatomy (Blackmore 1989) to make sense of what has been removed during an operation. The following are guidelines for talking with patients admitted for surgery.

- Ask for their understanding about why they are having surgery.
- Ask about their understanding of the name, location and function of the organ to be operated on.
- Ask them if they wish to know more about what will happen to them during and after surgery. Some people only want procedural information such as when they will be starved before they go to the operating theatre. Others will want more detailed information about drips and drains.
- Use simple diagrams to explain the location of organs.
- Talk through with them the meaning of any possible changes to their body. Do not make assumptions that everyone feels the same way about a similar operation. For example, some women perceive mastectomy to be a positive way to remove all their cancer, while others regard it as a severe form of mutilation (Fallowfield and Clark 1991).

- Remember that the way you react to patients with disfigurements may be incorporated by them into their self concept.
- Remember the range of social roles that people play forms their self concept. In hospital, we are unlikely to provide adequate opportunities for people to act out all their social roles, thus we often have a somewhat one-sided view of people. Remember that being a patient is also a social role.

Summary

- Children appear to demonstrate a series of different stages in their understandings of health and illness.

- Children develop 'scripts' as a result of experience which enable them to cope with future similar situations.

- Self concept is composed of the self image and self-esteem.

- Body image is an individual's perception of their body as a physiological, psychological and sociocultural entity.

- Visible changes in actual body image may serve to stigmatize an individual in the eyes of others.

- Self-esteem is the evaluative component of the self.

Further reading

Bull, R. (1988) *The Social Psychology of Facial Disfigurement*. New York: Springer-Verlag.
Hayes, N. (1994) *Foundations of Psychology: An Introductory Text*. London: Routledge. Chapter 13.
Lawler, J. (1991) *Behind the Screens: Somology and the Problem of the Body*. London: Churchill Livingstone.
Price, B. (1990) *Body Image: Nursing Concepts and Care*. New York: Prentice-Hall.

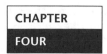

THEORIES OF LEARNING:
DEVELOPMENTS AND APPLICATIONS

Introduction

The purpose of this chapter and Chapter 5 is to introduce the new reader
to current psychological theories related to learning, perception and

memory. This chapter focuses upon selected aspects of learning theory which have proved to be of direct relevance to our understanding of health-related behaviours, including mental health. Students are encouraged to turn to basic introductory psychology texts for a more detailed theoretical account where appropriate.

Background to the development of learning theories

As a background to understanding current theories of learning, it is useful to gain some insight into the thinking which has influenced them. Prior to the nineteenth century, there existed a belief that knowledge was acquired by association because objects or situations were similar in some way (*similarity*), or because events occurred together at the same time or in the same place (*contiguity*), or through a relationship of *cause and effect*.

Psychologists have traditionally divided themselves into two camps. Those who believe that we are born *tabula rasa* (literally blank slate) and that all knowledge stems from experience are called **empiricists**. The **behaviourist** school of psychology is firmly rooted in the empiricist tradition. Behaviourists, with encouragement from Darwin's theory of evolution, make no distinction between the processes of animal and human learning, and claim that theories gained from animal studies can be applied to humans. They claim that the only legitimate way to demonstrate learning is to show a measurable association between the presentation of a **stimulus** (originally defined as something which excites sensory receptors, including vision, hearing, touch, smell or taste) and an observable response to it. Radical behaviourists actually believe that all behaviour is a function of external stimuli and not of internal thought processes (beliefs or intentions). They do not deny the existence of thought processes, but claim that these are 'private events' which cannot be studied directly and have no relevance to our understanding of the causes of human behaviour.

Exercise

How does the behaviourist view of causes of health-related behaviours, such as eating cream cakes, differ from the social cognition models outlined in Chapter 2? As you read on, consider the implications of behaviourist theories for health education.

The other main group of psychologists are the **nativists**. They believe that humans are born with unique abilities to structure knowledge in a special way. One of the main sources of support for the nativist view is the speed at which small children pick up language and learn to apply rules of grammar at a very early age. The study of thought processes (**cognition**) is central to the nativist tradition, since they believe that behaviour is determined by the way we think and process information. Some of these cognitive processes are examined in more detail in Chapter 5.

The argument between these two groups is not entirely resolved, although recent research suggests that behavioural and cognitive theories may not be as contradictory as was previously thought. Furthermore, it is not necessary to claim that one group is right and the other wrong in order to make good use of theories from both camps in the context of health care.

Behaviourist learning theories and behaviourism

Two of the best known behavioural theories, which were introduced in Chapter 1, are those of classical and operant (or instrumental) conditioning. **Conditioning** is a simple form of associative learning in which the response of an organism is shaped and maintained through pairing with an external stimulus. For this reason, it is sometimes referred to as S–R (stimulus–response) theory.

Classical conditioning

One of the first researchers to study animal behaviour, at the turn of the century, was Ivan Pavlov, who formulated the principle of **classical conditioning** from his famous studies with dogs. Dogs, like humans, salivate when they see food. This is a natural reflex response. Thus food is an unconditioned stimulus and salivation is an unconditioned (unlearned) response. Pavlov demonstrated that if a bell was consistently rung immediately prior to presenting the dog with food, the dog would eventually salivate as soon as the bell was rung, and before the food was seen. Salivation to a bell is not a natural, but a conditioned, reflex. Thus the bell is a conditioned stimulus and salivation to a bell is a conditioned response. This type of classical conditioning, or reflex learning, takes place without awareness, at a subconscious level.

Conditioned reflex responses

There are two important points to remember when applying the principle of classical conditioning:

1 All autonomic responses (those involving the arousal of the autonomic nervous system) are capable of conditioning by this type of association. Consider asthma, which is often caused by the constriction of the bronchus in response to an allergen. If a child has an allergic reaction to cat fur, it is possible that the child may, eventually, only have to see a cat in the distance to develop an asthma attack. Sometimes, these types of reflex responses may be generalized to pictures of cats or even other animals.

2 A conditioned reflex, like any reflex, is not normally under voluntary control. In the above example, asthma sufferers may be unaware that an asthma attack can be triggered in this way. Another example of a

conditioned reflex response is that of the nausea felt by cancer patients during courses of drug treatment and radiotherapy. Some eventually experience feelings of nausea as they approach the hospital, or even when they just think about the clinic. In other words, anything associated with the hospital is a conditioned stimulus and nausea has become a conditioned response.

Exercise

Think of other symptoms related to the autonomic nervous system which might be subject to classical conditioning and explain how these may have been acquired.

Conditioned emotional responses

Classical conditioning theory has helped us to understand the development of many fears and phobias. John Watson, a founding father of **behaviourism**, was able to demonstrate that a small child, called Little Albert, who showed no previous fear of any animal, developed a fear of white rats after a period in which the rat was presented to the child at the same time as a loud frightening noise (see Watson and Rayner 1920, in Gross 1994: ch. 16). Little Albert subsequently showed a fear of anything which was white and furry (this is termed **generalization**).

Most associations take repeated experiences to develop. However, one pairing with a strong autonomic arousal response can sometimes be enough to develop a conditioned fear response. For example, someone who has survived a coach accident may be too scared to get into any type of moving transport afterwards, even though they are aware that the chance of it happening again is extremely remote.

The principle of classical conditioning can account for fear of doctors, hospitals or medical equipment. For example, a child who has received a painful injection may later show fear of anyone in a white coat or any clinical situation. The mother and the staff may be unaware of the reason for this and feel that the child is behaving irrationally or just badly.

Exercise

Think of other situations where a patient's fear or anxiety might have been caused through classical conditioning and describe what effect this has on their current behaviour.

Undoing classically conditioned responses

Reasonable or rational argument will often not work for someone whose responses are classically conditioned. In fact fears, anxieties and phobias acquired in this way are often described as 'irrational' when the individual apparently knows that there is no reason to be afraid in the present circumstances, but still cannot control it. The most common way individuals deal with situations which cause fear or anxiety is to avoid them. However, **avoidance** is usually maladaptive, since it tends to perpetuate the problem. Agoraphobia is a fear of open spaces which causes people not to leave the house. The avoidance of going out can lead to crippling social consequences.

There are some therapeutic ways of dealing with these problems that health care professionals could benefit from knowing about, although expert help from a psychologist, or special training in these techniques, may be required.

1 Extinction

Once a conditioned stimulus is no longer associated with the unconditioned stimulus, the conditioned response fades and is eventually eliminated. For example, when the bell no longer signalled food for Pavlov's dogs, they eventually stopped salivating to the bell. The use of anti-nausea drugs by cancer patients in preparation for hospital attendance will stop the association of hospital with nausea and eventually eliminate the conditioned nausea response.

2 Counter-conditioning

Counter-conditioning implies the substitution of a negative conditioned response with a positive or non-harmful one. For example, full relaxation is a response which opposes the arousal of the autonomic nervous system and can be used to eliminate conditioned fear or anxiety responses. Once an individual has identified the stimulus which is triggering the problem, it may be possible to learn to substitute relaxation as a response. It should be noted that relaxation is a skill which takes time and perseverance to learn and use successfully.

3 Biofeedback

This involves the use of any kind of sensor which picks up autonomic activity such as moisture or temperature change, or muscular tension, and feeds it back as a continuous but variable audible signal (like a metal detector). This feedback can enable an individual to bring what is normally an automatic reflex under voluntary control. We often find it difficult to relax because we have no means of judging how successful we have been in relaxing tense muscles. The positioning of electrodes over an area of muscle will pick up the electrical activity of muscle contraction and allow it to be converted into an audible signal. As we relax, the signal changes. Once complete relaxation is achieved, the signal disappears altogether. This feedback makes it much easier to learn to relax fully.

4 Flooding

This can be used to treat fears and phobias. The individual is forcibly exposed to the situation or object they fear until the fear response has completely subsided. Flooding has been proved successful in eliminating a variety of fears and phobias, including fear of spiders. However, it needs great care as the individual may initially be very distressed. It is possible that an association, such as a conditioned fear response, may return after a long period of lack of exposure due to spontaneous recovery.

5 Systematic desensitization (Wolpe 1958)

This is a gentler approach to the treatment for anxieties and phobias. People are first taught relaxation techniques to counter their normal autonomic stress response. They then learn to apply the relaxation technique in a 'hierarchical' series of graded situations from imagining a mild fear-producing situation to imagining a more severe fear-producing situation, to looking at pictures or films, to approaching the actual situation, to actual exposure. At each stage, the individual must demonstrate control through relaxation before proceeding to the next stage. Wolpe also recommended assertiveness training (training people to stand up for themselves) as an additional means of helping them to gain control over anxiety-provoking social encounters. Systematic desensitization is time-consuming but has proved successful in treating a wide variety of incapacitating and long-standing conditioned emotional responses.

Exercise

Think back to your example of a patient whose anxiety or fear was caused through classical conditioning. Consider how any of the above techniques might be useful in helping to reduce or eliminate this response. How might you set about this?

The importance of fear-reduction in hospital settings

Classically conditioned emotional responses are often troublesome and difficult to treat. It is far better to avoid conditioned fear responses in hospital settings in the first place through adequate preparation. One important way in which people differ from other animals is that we can communicate with each other. Therefore, nurses and therapists can help patients to anticipate potentially frightening stimuli (injections, procedures, etc.) so that they do not experience sudden autonomic arousal.

Exercise

Can you think of any other examples of the application of conditioning principles in the prevention or treatment of other problems related to health or social care?

A good example of a treatment which is directly derived from conditioning principles is the bell and pad, which is used to stop bed-wetting in older children. The theory is that the bell sounds as soon as urine touches the pad and wakes the child up to get out to the toilet. The bell prompts the association of urination with wakening, which eventually leads the child to wake and go to the toilet when there is a desire to urinate. In reality, in the initial stages, it is often the bell which wakes the parent who then wakes the sleeping child. Therefore, the successful application of this technique usually depends upon the cooperation and perseverance of the parents!

Operant (instrumental) conditioning

Operant conditioning refers to behavioural learning which takes place as a result of the consequences or outcomes of voluntary (as opposed to reflex) behaviour. Operant theory was a move away from the S–R approach. Operant conditioning theory proposes that behavioural learning takes place as a result of **reinforcement** and **punishment**. For example, I learn from experience that eating strawberries is pleasurable so I eat more. In this case, the strawberry is termed a **reinforcer** because it increases the likelihood that my behaviour (eating them) will be repeated. Or, I learn that if I touch a hot iron I will burn myself so I don't touch it again. Here the hot iron is termed a **punisher** because it decreases the likelihood that I will repeat the action.

Anything which fulfils basic needs, such as food, drink and sex, is termed a **primary reinforcer**. A substance such as nicotine may be regarded as a primary reinforcer once an individual has become dependent on it. A **secondary reinforcer** is one which is related to primary reinforcement. For example, money can be traded to gain primary reinforcers. Social approval or praise is a powerful source of secondary reinforcement in human society, whereas the social disapproval of a peer group or 'significant other' is a powerful source of punishment.

The psychologist famous for the development of the principles of operant conditioning was B.F. Skinner. These principles have been derived from the animal laboratory using such equipment as the 'Skinner box', in which a light or sound is used to signal to the animal or bird that, if it presses a lever or pecks a key, it will receive a food reward. Thus animals have been trained to respond to different types of stimulus or cue and the effect on the animal's behaviour of different patterns or **schedules of reinforcement** have been measured. Only principles which are thought to be most useful in health care practice are referred to here, and the reader is encouraged to refer to a general psychology text for a more detailed account of reinforcement theory.

Discriminative stimuli (cues)

Individuals quickly learn that certain actions only lead to desired consequences under certain conditions or in certain contexts. For example, red traffic lights signal stop, whereas green traffic lights signal go. Discriminative cues are not always obvious. For example, a mother may express disapproval, or even smack a very young child for going near a fire. This may stop the child from doing this in her presence and she might assume that it is now safe to leave the child alone in the room with the fire switched on. However, in the absence of the discriminative stimulus (in this case the mother), the child may approach and touch the fire.

Many behaviours which influence health are referred to as being under **stimulus control**. For example, the smoker may respond automatically to a cup of coffee by lighting up a cigarette.

Schedules of reinforcement or punishment

Sometimes, an occasional or intermittent strong reward can reinforce behaviour more strongly than continuous small rewards. Gambling is a good example of how one large win (or even the possibility of a large win) can provide strong motivation to continue for a very long time. In fact, continuous reinforcement may lead to satiation. For example, if we always praise people, it is eventually taken for granted and ceases to affect their performance. An occasional stiff speeding penalty may be sufficient to reduce driving speed.

The nature and strength of reinforcement and punishment is subjective

Reinforcement is not necessarily the same thing as reward. Food is only reinforcing if I am hungry and I like the food on offer. Some children who receive little adult attention may behave badly to provoke punishment as a source of attention. In these circumstances, the punishment is actually a reinforcer of behaviour.

Smoking may seem disgusting to a non-smoker, but it has a number of highly reinforcing consequences to a smoker which need to be taken into account if the smoker is to stop.

The immediacy of the consequence

Generally, the more immediate the consequence, the more powerful the effect. Small children will normally take a small chocolate bar now, rather than wait for a large one later (if they like chocolate). We can learn to **delay gratification** through experience, but the effect of an immediate reward is still very powerful. Many people who really want to lose weight in the longer term find it impossible to resist the immediate satisfaction of eating something now.

Punishment frequently fails to work because it is administered long after the crime was committed and the association between the crime and the punishment is therefore weakened. However, some types of consequence do not lose their impact by delay. For example, experiments have shown that rats made ill by poison will subsequently avoid the type of food or drink that contained the poison, even when there is a substantial delay between eating the food and being ill (Garcia *et al.* 1966, in Gross 1994: ch. 31). This type of association clearly has survival value and has given rise to the theory that some responses are innately primed or **prepared**.

The certainty of the consequences

In order to have any impact on behaviour, the reinforcing or punishing consequences must be either certain to occur or, if uncertain, be more likely than unlikely. Another reason why punishment fails to eliminate or reduce crime is because the chances of getting caught are not very great.

Healthy people often don't take preventive health advice because they have never experienced a direct relationship between cause (their behaviour) and consequence (becoming ill). This may explain why many people fail to take action until symptoms become apparent (often too late).

Replacement activity

Behaviours play an important role in filling time in our lives, in addition to producing desirable outcomes. Therefore, if someone wishes to give up one behaviour, it is necessary to replace it with something else which is equally rewarding and occupies as much time.

Drinking eight pints of beer is not only satisfying to the taste and the thirst, it is usually a relaxing social activity which occupies a whole evening in the pub. To give up or cut down drinking will require finding something else which provides the same amount of social relaxation. Drinking low-alcohol lager or a soft drink will generally serve that function, provided it gains the social approval of one's drinking companions.

Avoidance

Avoidance is a common response to punishment but, as has been pointed out, it is not always adaptive. One of the most common primary sources of punishment is pain. Pain can occur as a consequence of tissue damage caused by accident or disease or it can be inflicted by others. Escape or avoidance behaviours are adaptive responses to accidental pain, since they remove us from the cause and ensure that we avoid future exposure to painful stimuli. However, in chronic pain it can lead to a reduction in all forms of activity which persists after the pain has actually subsided.

Monitoring the ABC (antecedents – behaviour – consequences)

Behaviourists recommend that before any programme of behaviour change is started (for example, helping someone to give up smoking or eliminate their child's temper tantrums, or reduce anxiety), the frequency of the behaviour should be recorded, together with its *immediate* causes and consequences. This is termed **functional analysis** of behaviour. The frequency of the behaviour provides a baseline from which to judge success. The causes and consequences identify sources of stimulus control, together with sources of reinforcement and punishment. These can then be altered in order to modify behaviour.

The immediate causes and consequences are not always what they seem. For example, the mother may be unaware that the reason why her child has so many tantrums is because they always result in her giving the child attention. This can be identified using a simple diary (see Westmacott and Cameron 1981). Providing attention when a child is being good and withdrawing attention when a child behaves badly to attract attention quickly reduces attention-seeking behaviour and is a technique used successfully by teachers in the classroom.

Behaviour modification

Behaviour modification refers to the changing of behaviour through the deliberate manipulation of sources of reinforcement which are normally controlled by another person or persons. Behaviour modification is based directly upon Skinnerian operant principles.

Behaviour modification was popular in controlling socially undesirable or obsessive behaviours in long-stay mental illness institutions using a **token economy** (Ayllon and Azrin 1968). Socially desirable behaviours were reinforced by immediately giving tokens which could be exchanged for primary reinforcers of the patient's choice (sadly, this often took the form of cigarettes). Antisocial behaviour was ignored (not punished).

Behaviour modification has also proved useful for reinforcing socially desirable behaviour in children (in the home and in the classroom), and in people with learning difficulties. Punishment is not part of this regime and undesirable behaviours are usually ignored. 'Time out' (e.g. leaving the room) may be necessary to isolate uncontrollable individuals for short periods until they have calmed down, but early distraction into alternative desirable behaviours which are then rewarded by praise or a prize is generally a more successful approach.

Exercise

Behaviour modification has been used as another approach to curing bed-wetting for children who are capable of achieving bladder control. Can you identify a method of incentive which might be suitable as a reward for having a dry bed? How might you put this into operation? (see Westmacott and Cameron)

Overlearning (habit formation)

When we initially learn a new skill, we tend to break it down into a series of simple steps and learn each one in turn. Therefore, learning is initially slow. As we become more proficient, we are able to act faster and perform certain steps or sequences 'without thinking'. This is how we learn to drive a car or give an injection. Eventually, all the actions which make up the skill are integrated and performed 'automatically'. This is termed **overlearning**. Behaviours which are overlearned are usually never forgotten (you don't forget how to ride a bike). When sequences of everyday behaviour are overlearned, we call them **habits**.

Overlearning helps to explain why some health-related behaviours are difficult to start or very hard to stop. Taking up a new behaviour, such as exercise or relaxation, is unlikely to be maintained until we no longer have to think about doing it. Conversely, overlearned habits, such as poor posture, will be difficult to stop, even when the individual knows that they are bad for health.

Problems with behaviourism

Behaviourist principles have proved fruitful in many areas of health care and can be judged by their usefulness. However, behaviourism has become less popular with psychologists and the public in recent years for a number of reasons. The public have become unhappy about the use of animals in any type of experimentation. Many psychologists reject behaviourism because it appears to contradict the notion of free will, denies the uniqueness of the human being, and may not be applicable to complex human thought and behaviour. Skinner himself believed that the principles of operant conditioning applied equally to humans as to animals and was very humane in his own applications of these principles. For example, he highlighted the ethical and practical problems associated with punishment and suggested that human behaviour should be regulated only by reinforcement and not by punishment. He acknowledged that it would be difficult to determine how any organism might respond to a particular situation in real life because their response is likely to be determined by the sum of their reinforcement histories (past experiences). Animal subjects of conditioning experiments have to be kept from birth in unstimulating environments to ensure that their responses are not affected by previous experiences. However, there remain doubts that learning occurs only as a result of direct experience and these are considered below as a matter of interest.

As early as the 1920s, Kohler's famous studies of chimpanzees indicated that some novel behaviours involve deliberation or 'insight'. For example, chimpanzees when faced with a banana which was out of reach were observed to study the situation and then pile boxes on top of each other to reach the banana, even though they had never done this before. Harlow's subsequent observations of chimpanzees indicated that they acquired this ability through applying strategies which they had learned from previous experiences in different situations. Harlow termed this a 'learning set' or learning how to learn. It appears that even animals are able to predict a successful course of action by integrating knowledge gained from a variety of past experiences.

Another problem which still causes heated debate among psychologists is the way that language is learned. Most people would agree that the acquisition of language is not primarily dependent upon external reinforcement, although others would argue that verbal behaviour is used to gain primary or secondary reinforcement and point to the fact that chimpanzees have been taught to use sign language creatively through the use of reinforcement (Gardner and Gardner 1969, in Gross 1994: ch. 28). Noam Chomsky has frequently and vehemently argued that behaviourist principles are not adequate to account for the speed with which language is initially learned by children, nor for the application of grammatical rules. He has adopted a nativist view and proposed the existence of a specific 'language acquisition device' which is unique to humans. There appear to be problems with each of these extreme (empiricist *vs* nativist) views and neither can be said yet to have won this debate.

Cognitive reinterpretation of conditioning theories

Although behaviourism is regarded with scepticism by many people nowadays, behavioural psychology has continued to produce exciting results since the 1970s. Researchers working within the behavioural tradition of animal experimentation have been able to make inferences about the cognitive (thought) processes which underlie 'conditioned' responses and this has prompted them to reinterpret conditioning processes. This work not only provides a direct link between behavioural and cognitive psychology, but has shed some light on the nature of information processing. It has led to the comment that learning theorists are 'all cognitivists now'. One of the main advances of contemporary learning theory has been in identifying and understanding the importance of prediction and control. These concepts are central to health psychology and are considered below. Many of these aspects are taken up again in Chapter 6 to understand stress and coping.

Probability learning and predictability

Based upon more recent behavioural experimentation, it has been possible to account for both classical and operant conditioning, not in terms of the pairing of stimulus and response, but in terms of the ability of an organism (whether human or otherwise) to predict the probability of events or outcomes occurring, on the basis of prior experiences in the same or similar situations. Thus in Pavlov's experiment on classical conditioning, it is the power of the bell to predict food which determines salivation, and not an S–R association. Likewise in operant conditioning, it is the predictive power of the cue, together with the predicted consequences, which are important in determining the response.

The child in the room with the fire may be said to have predicted, from experience, that it is not wise to go near the fire when mummy is around or she will be angry. This implies that it is OK to touch the fire when mummy cannot see. The child may not yet have experienced or understood the relationship between cause (touching the fire) and effect (getting burned). Examples such as this do not necessarily imply that conscious thought processes are taking place. Much of this type of 'information processing' takes place automatically at a subconscious level and it would be a mistake to assume that the child's actions are either a deliberate act of defiance or the result of stupidity.

Demonstrating that animals can predict the probability of outcomes in simple laboratory situations does not necessarily imply that this explains complex learning. Nevertheless, if it can be demonstrated that it is possible to generate transferable predictive rules from past experience, it is possible that this simple cognitive principle could be used to account for both the 'insightful' learning demonstrated by Kohler's monkeys and the child's ability to generate grammatical rules during language development. This would draw contemporary behavioural and cognitive psychology even closer together.

The importance of predictability has proved influential in health settings and is demonstrated by research into preparation for potentially painful medical and surgical procedures (see also Chapter 6). If the patient, whether a child or an adult, is given no warning, the sudden pain can lead to strong autonomic arousal. This can cause a conditioned fear response which may subsequently generalize to a variety of medical situations. A warning can act as a **safety signal**. It arouses anxiety throughout the procedure, but sudden autonomic response is not triggered. Events for which we are prepared are much easier to tolerate than unexpected events and do not normally lead to any lasting damage. The explanation appears to lie in the degree of control we perceive ourselves to have over events or situations.

Loss of control, learned helplessness and depression

An important contribution to applied health and clinical psychology, which originated in the animal behaviour laboratory in the 1960s, was the concept of **learned helplessness**, which was formulated by Martin Seligman and his colleagues (see Seligman 1975). Two dogs were administered an identical series of minor electric shocks. One dog was provided with the means to terminate the shock by pressing a panel with its muzzle. Not only did this dog learn to avoid the shock, but was quickly able to learn to avoid subsequent shocks when transferred to a different environment, a 'shuttle box', where it had to jump over a small barrier to escape. The other dog received exactly the same shocks at the same time as the first dog but had no control over them. When transferred to the shuttle box this dog did not attempt to escape. This dog showed a motivational deficit (it made no attempt to move), it showed a cognitive deficit (it failed to recognize a simple escape route) and it showed an emotional deficit (it appeared very miserable). The differences in the behaviours of the two dogs could only be attributable to the level of control each had in the first situation, and not to the shock received. The first dog was 'in control' and therefore expected to have control in subsequent situations. The second dog had no control and learned to predict that it had no subsequent control.

According to Seligman, learned helplessness means learning that one's own actions have no influence upon outcomes. He noted that these motivational, cognitive and emotional deficits are all symptomatic of human depression. He and his colleagues later found that the 'helpless' dog lost these symptoms only after the experimenter had physically dragged it across the barrier on numerous occasions to demonstrate that it was possible to regain control and escape the shock. When applied to human depression, this suggests that depressed individuals must relearn, through personal experience, that they are capable of doing something positive to influence what happens in their lives. It is not sufficient to tell someone that, of course, they could do it if they tried. It is necessary to identify the skills available to the individual and then engage them in tasks where success is assured. In this way, they learn, through experience, that they can regain control.

Lack of control over their lives has been suggested as one reason to account for the higher incidence of depression among the unemployed, those on low pay, those with less education, and women. Mirowsky and Ross (1989) demonstrated that depression among these groups is caused by the reality of their circumstances and not by personal depressive tendencies which have brought them down the social scale. This being so, it is probably more helpful to encourage them to increase their sense of power by joining self-help or pressure groups, than by focusing upon personal inadequacies.

The work on controllability versus uncontrollability has practical implications well beyond the understanding and treatment of human depression. Subsequent experiments with humans into perceived control over outcomes suggest that when individuals believe that they have control over aversive stimuli, such as noise or discomfort, they are able to tolerate much higher levels than if they believe they have no control. This explains why we enjoy the fresh air when we open the window, but complain about the draught when someone else does!

Predictability and controllability are closely linked. If I cannot predict what is going to happen, I am unlikely to be able to control it. This is why the giving of information to patients is so important. As one elderly gentleman commented: 'You can only deal with what you know about'. However, predicting what will happen does not guarantee that an individual will know how to handle the situation. Therefore, information about what patients can do to help themselves in a particular situation is as important as information about what will happen. This may involve teaching coping skills; for example, learning to feed a baby, by any method, takes a certain amount of skill on the part of the mother and some guidance will help. Quite often, patients are left feeling helpless because we take it for granted that they know what to do and how to do it, when they do not. It is also important to ensure that patients know how to summon help when they no longer feel in control of the situation, particularly in a hospital situation where they do not have full control themselves.

Exercise

Consider elderly patients who are being looked after in an institutional setting. What factors are likely to make them feel helpless? What effect might this have on them? How might they be helped to feel more in control? Why is this a good thing?

Langer and Rodin (1976) demonstrated that elderly people living in institutional care who were given a greater say in decision making, more control over their environment and increased personal responsibility, such as having a plant to look after, showed greater levels of activity, were happier and tended to live longer than those who had no control. The issue of control is examined further in Chapter 6, which examines stress and coping with hospitalization.

Social learning theory

It is self-evident that the majority of human learning takes place in a social environment and not, as in animal experiments, in an isolated environment. This raises important questions about whether social behaviour involves the same learning processes, or if social learning is quite different. It appears that there are both similarities and differences. One of the main differences is that social learning can take place by imitation.

Observational learning

One of the greatest originators and current proponents of social learning theory is Albert Bandura. Bandura emerged from the behaviourist tradition, but was critical of Skinner's assertions that human behaviour is passively driven by external cues and consequences, although he continued to acknowledge that these are influential. He conducted a series of classic experiments during the 1960s which clearly showed that children don't just learn from the consequences of their own actions. They are capable of **modelling** their behaviour on that of others and are capable of judging the likely consequences of their own actions by observing the consequences for others of their actions (**vicarious reinforcement**). His experiments in which children imitated, without prompting or incentive, aggressive adult behaviour towards a 'Bobo' doll (Bandura et al. 1961, in Gross 1994: ch. 14), raised fears about the possibility that children mimic aggressive or violent behaviour seen on television.

Bandura's work on modelling or imitative learning helps to fill in some of the gaps in explaining the learning of language. Babies are able to imitate facial expressions and movements within the first days of life and recent research has demonstrated that they imitate and rehearse sounds long before they make their first meaningful word. This is why hearing, and hence hearing testing, is important at a very early stage of language development.

Work on the importance of modelling in social learning suggests that parents and health professionals should act as role models in relation to health. There is evidence that children are more likely to smoke if their parents smoke. 'Do as I say, not as I do' is just not good enough.

Exercise

Think of as many health-related and illness-related behaviours as you can (good and bad ones) which might have been learned through modelling. In what ways do you think that role models could be used in the promotion of health? Do you think that health professionals should act as role models for healthy living?

Self-efficacy and self-esteem

Bandura went on to propose that once children have learned to imitate any new skill, such as the use of language, they are quite capable of monitoring and adjusting their own performance through a process of self-regulation, by comparing their own performance with that of others. Through this active process, they achieve a sense of **self-efficacy** (personal competence or mastery), which leads to a sense of **self-esteem** (feelings of personal worth). Bandura argued that we actually reward ourselves for a good performance, while the failure to recognize and reward ourselves for good performance can lead to depression. Bandura suggested that talented people often become depressed because they set themselves standards of achievement which are too high.

The principles of behaviour modification can be used to help anyone change their behaviour through **self-modification**. They should first monitor the causes, consequences and frequency of their own behaviour and then take steps to alter their routine in order to change regular cues, or provide themselves with treats or self-praise to reinforce successful behaviour and boost self-esteem. This may all require a little guidance or encouragement from health professionals or therapists.

It is interesting to note that Bandura's account of the development of self-esteem is somewhat similar to that of the humanist psychologists. Bandura proposes that self-esteem is a result of satisfaction with our own performance. Humanists have suggested that self-esteem reflects a close fit between what we believe ourselves to be and what we would like to be. Social comparison is important to both theories in determining what a 'good' or 'acceptable' performance should be. Self-esteem may be lost if we set ourselves unrealistic targets.

Exercise

Think of a skill you might wish to teach a patient in any setting. Describe how a knowledge of modelling, positive reinforcement and self-regulation might help you to formulate a teaching programme which will ensure that the patient achieves a sense of self-efficacy.

Learning to attribute causes in social situations: Locus of control

During the 1970s it was recognized that, although theories of learning which had been developed in the animal laboratory might have implications for human learning, the majority of human experience takes place in a social context where much of the reinforcement of behaviour is socially determined. Attribution theory proposes that we interpret things that happen to us according to three dimensions: (1) internal (it was my own actions) *vs* external (it was due to 'powerful others' or it was luck, fate or chance); (2) stable (I always make the same attribution in this situation) *vs* unstable (my attributions vary); and (3) global (I make this attribution in all situations) *vs* specific (I only make this attribution in this situation).

It has been found that **causal attributions** tend to be relatively stable over time and are used to make predictions about future actions and outcomes. A pattern of stable and global attributions may be regarded as a personality characteristic and is termed **locus of control**. People's attributions about health and the development of illness are termed **health locus of control** (HLOC; Wallston *et al.* 1978):

1 *Internal HLOC*. Individuals who have internal locus of control are likely to believe that health and recovery from illness are dependent upon their own actions. These people are most likely to initiate their own prevention or treatment programme, or to demand and use information which will enable them to take care of themselves (Peterson and Stunkard 1989).

2 *External (powerful others) HLOC*. People who attribute the responsibility for preventing or treating illness to 'powerful others' (such as doctors) are more likely to seek advice from a doctor when they have symptoms and may be more likely to take advice from a doctor when it is given (they are likely to do as they are told), but they may be less likely to initiate or sustain their own actions.

3 *External (luck, fate or chance) HLOC*. People who hold these attributions believe that the maintenance of health or the onset of illness is a matter of luck, fate or chance. They have little motivation to take any personal action and are unlikely to believe that others can do much to help.

A number of studies in a variety of primary and tertiary health care settings have indicated that individuals who have external (luck, fate or chance) HLOC are unlikely to take action to promote health or prevent illness or to take responsibility for actions which promote rehabilitation once they are ill (e.g. McLean and Pietroni 1990). Further illustrations of the relevance of beliefs in control are given in Chapters 6 and 8.

Bandura's concept of self-efficacy is closely linked to locus of control, such that those with a strong sense of perceived self-efficacy in relation to a range of tasks are likely to believe that their actions can have a positive influence on outcomes and demonstrate internal locus of control. These relationships are explored further in Chapter 6.

> **Exercise**
>
> An elderly man who lives alone has had a stroke which has left a slight weakness in his left arm (he is right-handed). He is undergoing rehabilitation prior to his return home. How can hospital staff apply learning and attribution theories to ensure that he is likely to undertake 'self-care' once he is home?

Causal attributions, learned helplessness and depression

Seligman and his colleagues proposed that people who are depressed tend to hold internal, stable and global attributions about negative outcomes. In other words, they attribute their misfortune to themselves and believe that it will always be like this in all situations. However, this proposition is contradicted by applied research which indicates that people who are depressed are more likely to have external (chance) locus of control. For example, Skevington (1983) found that people with rheumatoid arthritis are more likely to be depressed if they believe that neither they nor anyone else can do anything to help relieve their pain. This is termed **universal helplessness** and is associated with feelings of hopelessness. You may find it useful to refer to Fig. 6.4 to help you to understand this further.

The origins of locus of control and related concepts

If internal or external expectations about future outcomes are based upon past experiences, then it seems logical to assume that childhood is an important period in the development of causal attributions. Parents provide the environment in which children begin to learn about how to deal with the world around them. Other influential external factors throughout childhood include experiences with teachers, peers and significant others. However, there is research evidence to link the child's locus of control with parenting style (Baumrind 1967). Warm-directive, or authoritative, is used to describe the parent who maintains firm standards but provides reasons for discipline, encourages personal responsibility, and gives positive and negative feedback in an atmosphere of 'positive regard'. This style is more likely to help shape an individual with internal locus of control, high self-esteem and self-confidence. Authoritarian parenting (strong parental control) is associated with a lack of independence, external (powerful others) locus of control, low self-esteem and a lack of affection towards others (this may imply that they are poor at providing emotional support to others).

The importance of social skills

Each individual is born with an individual personality which is likely to shape their interaction with the people around them. A smile from a baby acts as a powerful reinforcer for the mother to feed and protect it. This in turn reinforces the child's own responses. Social behaviour is learned through all of the processes identified above: through classically conditioned reflexes, through primary and secondary reinforcement and punishment, through modelling, through vicarious reinforcement or punishment (watching other being rewarded or punished for certain actions), through predicting outcomes and through self-regulation and monitoring.

Since social approval is one of the main sources of reinforcement in our lives, it is evident that those likely to gain most of this type of reinforcement are those who have outgoing and sociable personalities and have learned good social or interpersonal skills.

One theory of depression put forward by Lewinsohn (1974) proposed that individuals become depressed because they lack the ability to gain positive reinforcement from other people because of a lack of social skills. Certainly, some mentally ill people are singled out because of their 'odd' or socially unacceptable behaviour and this leads other people to avoid them. These people may be particularly noticeable on our streets at the present time because of the closure of long-stay mental institutions. Social skills training is an important component of therapy and rehabilitation for people with depression, since this enables them to gain social acceptance, which, in turn, increases their sense of self-efficacy and self-esteem.

Social skills training, together with positive reinforcement, is also an essential part of working with people who have learning disabilities because they find it difficult to identify non-verbal cues, or are unable to recognize, or imitate successfully, socially appropriate behaviour in a given set of circumstances.

Social skills are important for physical health as well as mental health, since they enable individuals to gain social support from friends and partners (see Chapter 6) and thus share health information and receive prompting to seek medical help when they need it.

A social cognitive–behavioural approach to assist someone to stop smoking, once they have decided that they wish to do so

The final section of this chapter will assist the reader in applying principles from behavioural, cognitive and social learning theories to help empower patients to change their behaviour. It is important that this programme is only targeted at those who have decided to change, but are finding it difficult to achieve this. Persuading them to give up in the first place is considered separately in Chapter 9. Smoking is used as the exemplar. The approach is based upon a successful programme devised by David Marks (1994).

First, it is necessary to take account of the following factors and share them with the patient:

1 Nicotine has positive (reinforcing) consequences for the smoker: it is relaxing, increases alertness and improves cognitive performance.

2 Because of these effects, smoking provides a useful way of coping with stress.
3 Smoking a cigarette fills time, provides thinking time for problem solving, and 'time out' from difficult situations.
4 Smoking provides something to do. Eating often replaces this, but leads to weight gain.
5 Many people relapse because they gain weight.
6 Smoking is a social activity (provides social reinforcement) and the smoker is often under peer pressure to smoke.
7 Lighting up is a habit which takes place in certain situations without thinking (e.g. having a cup of coffee or after a meal).

The following techniques address these points directly. Will-power is not an issue in this programme and the individual does not need to stop smoking from day one. Smoking behaviour declines naturally as the programme is implemented.

1 Interrupt the habit of taking out a cigarette by putting a rubber band round the packet which must first be removed.
2 Reduce the association of cigarettes with pleasure: place a personal message under the rubber band and read it out each time a cigarette is drawn out. For example, 'This cigarette is making me ill. I do not like this cigarette. I do not wish to smoke this cigarette'. The individual *must* then take out a cigarette and smoke it so that an association is built up between the cigarette and something unpleasant.
3 Reduce the habitual effect by identifying the situations in which the patient tends to light up without thinking by placing another message under the rubber band to read out before lighting the cigarette in that situation: 'Just because I have had a meal, I do not need to smoke. Next time I have finished a meal, I will not want to smoke'.
4 Find new ways of keeping the hands occupied, such as doodling (the Greeks use worry beads).
5 Build in an exercise and weight-control programme to prevent excessive weight gain.
6 Rehearse assertive skills for saying 'no' to peers.
7 Find social support from others who do not smoke.
8 Find alternative methods of stress management (e.g. relaxation, yoga).

The following abbreviated case study provides an example of how this can be applied.

Case study: Pam

Pam is a married woman aged 40. She has severe Raynaud's disease, which has already led to the amputation of the tops of her left fingers. She also had a stroke which has left a weakness on her right (dominant) side and a speech impediment which is worse when she is anxious. She knows that her health problems are due to smoking but has failed many times to give up. She has always had a lot of problems with her 'nerves'. She now sits at home all day doing nothing but watch television and feels helpless and hopeless. Her husband is very attentive, does all the housework and prepares all their meals. The doctor has advised her that giving up smoking is the only way of improving her condition and that there is nothing more he can do until she has stopped. Pam wept and her husband became angry. What can they do?

At first glance, the situation appeared somewhat hopeless. However, it emerged that there are many aspects of her situation which could be addressed to improve her quality of life, even if she is unable to stop smoking completely. The first thing was to acknowledge that smoking gives her a sense of well-being and is not something that she could be expected to give up 'just like that'. This made Pam and her husband more willing to discuss the situation.

It emerged that she smokes her first cigarette on waking every morning and only after that experiences severe pain in her left hand. Therefore, Pam's message for her cigarette packet states that 'this cigarette will cause me excruciating pain'. Pam was encouraged to change her daily routine by removing some of the cues that trigger lighting up a cigarette. For example, she would start by leaving her cigarettes downstairs at night and spend more time in the bathroom before going down to make herself some breakfast in the morning. Since her husband did not smoke, there was little temptation to smoke socially.

Pam needs some kind of occupation during the daytime and thought that, in spite of her pain and disability, she could take up crochet again and would enjoy that. Stroking and talking to the dog is another activity which is also enjoyable and stress-reducing. Her husband does so much for her because he wants to feel helpful, but agreed it would be better to do less and encourage her to do as much as she can around the house. Pam could also take the dog for regular short walks, initially under his supervision, to exercise and meet other people casually without any initial pressure to speak to them.

The need to replace the stress-reducing effects of smoking were discussed. Pam enjoyed attending yoga classes in the past and found them helpful. Although she has lost the confidence to attend a group, she felt she would like to practise yoga and relaxation at home, using a tape to help her. Pam finally agreed to monitor the number of cigarettes she smokes and record the situations which prompt her to smoke, but no targets were set for reduction.

This programme does *not* rely upon will-power but aims to build up a sense of self-efficacy. It provides a positive action plan in which failure is not a component, since although smoking reduction would be a desirable outcome, it is not the primary focus. Instead of feeling a victim of herself, Pam began to feel that there are things that she can both enjoy and succeed at. Since these activities are built upon existing skills, they reinforce her sense of self-efficacy and increase her self-esteem. The programme encourages her to take personal control and stop relying solely upon her husband. The activities discussed are all designed to improve her quality of life, quite apart from helping her to reduce her cigarette consumption.

She went away from the initial one-hour consultation smiling and appearing a little more self-confident. Later consultations would focus upon building up Pam's sense of self-efficacy and encouraging her husband to do likewise. This example illustrates how behavioural learning principles can be incorporated into a cognitive programme which utilizes a patient-centred approach and humanistic aims.

Summary

- Behavioural theories of learning are based upon the belief that observable behaviour is a function of environmental stimuli and consequences.

- Classical conditioning theory may help to explain the development of fears and phobias and can be used to treat these.

- The principles of operant conditioning explain behaviour in terms of experiences of reinforcement and punishment in different contexts.

- Behaviourist learning theories have been redefined in cognitive terms, with particular reference to predictability.

- Learned helplessness (uncontrollability) has been proposed as a model for understanding human depression.

- Social learning theory adds to the understanding of learning through observing and modelling behaviour on that of other people.

- Individuals learn to attribute outcomes to themselves, others, or chance. Stable attributions are termed locus of control.

- Social skills are an important factor in determining self-efficacy and self-esteem.

- A cognitive–behavioural programme to assist people who have decided to stop smoking is presented and illustrated.

Further reading

Atkinson, R.L., Atkinson, R.C., Smith, E.E. and Bem, D.J. (1993) *Introduction to Psychology*, 11th edn. Orlando, FL: Harcourt Brace Jovanovich. Chapter 7.

Bandura, A.A. (1977) *Social Learning Theory*. Englewood Cliffs, NJ: Prentice-Hall.

Gross, R.D. (1994) *Key Studies in Psychology*, 2nd edn. London: Hodder and Stoughton. Chapters 14, 16, 28 and 31.

Mirowsky, J. and Ross, C.E. (1989) *Social Causes of Psychological Distress*. New York: Aldine de Gruyter.

Schaffer, D.R. (1988) *Social and Personality Development*, 2nd edn. Pacific Grove, CA: Brooks/Cole. Chapters 3 and 8.

Westmacott, E.V.S. and Cameron, R.J. (1981) *Behaviour Can Change*. London: Macmillan.

CHAPTER FIVE

PERCEPTION, MEMORY AND PATIENT INFORMATION-GIVING

Introduction

The previous chapter focused on the development of theories of learning and the gradual move from behaviourist theories, which made no assumptions about thought processes, to socio-cognitive theories with their emphasis upon attribution. This chapter will focus upon cognitive theories of perception and memory and will consider how these too have evolved from context-free research to research and applications in a social context.

Theories of perception

Perception is the process which determines the way we appraise the world around us and forms the basis of the actions we take to remain in control of what is going on in our lives. The significance of this will become more apparent in Chapter 6 on stress and coping. One of the main problems in considering psychological theories of perception is that they are usually presented in standard psychology texts in such a way as to reduce their apparent relevance to real-life situations such as health care. This chapter will focus upon both theories and applications.

Theories of sensory perception have traditionally focused upon visual perception because this has been an area of particular interest to researchers. Put in a simplistic way, the eye has long been regarded as similar to a camera in which an image of an external object is formed on the retina. This stimulates rods and cones which relay the image to the brain where a mental representation of the object is formed. This is called **representational theory**. According to Richard Gregory (1970; see Gross 1992), this representation is not an exact mirror of reality, but is a 'shorthand' interpretation of reality which is informed by past experience so that sensory material is reduced to something which is manageable and interpretable through a process of selectivity. During this process, ambiguities are unravelled, gaps are filled, and inferences about the visual image are made. Thus, according to this view, what we see is not reality, but our own interpretation of reality. An example of this is the way in which we judge distance and depth from the flat retinal image by learning to use visual cues. These include relative size and position of familiar objects, the distant convergence of straight lines and binocular disparity (the slight differences between the images at each eye).

Evidence in support of perception as a constructive process, as proposed within representational theory, takes the form of the visual illusion. Here the human eye is shown to make sense of something which is nonsense, or convert something which is incomplete into something which is complete or familiar in order to make sense of it. There are many persuasive examples of these in psychology textbooks which the student is encouraged to look at.

Opposition to representational theory has come from James Gibson (1966; see Gross 1992), who proposed the *theory of direct perception*. Gibson claimed that the brain has no need to construct a visual reality from limited flat visual images on the retina. His early work in aircraft landing simulation led him to assert that our visual interpretation of the world around us is based upon information which is contained in the rich flow of textured and structured light which moves across the retina as we move. Furthermore, he proposed that we actively seek to distinguish between things in our environment which are stable and things which are changing or new. Visual illusions rarely occur in the real world if we have unrestricted access and movement. In fact, visual illusions have to be carefully constructed to limit the amount of detail available on the page, or to restrict the viewpoint of the observer. A three-dimensional illusion is impossible to construct unless viewed through a pinhole. The first thing we normally do when faced with an ambiguous view is to move about to gain additional detail from different viewpoints.

Thus representational theory portrays humans as passive receivers of flat retinal images which are translated by the brain, while the theory of direct perception portrays humans as active seekers of information which is contained in the rich environmental sources available to us and re-quires no further interpretation.

The reality of perception is that we do not just rely upon one source of sensation in order to appraise what is going on. In addition to the visual system, we use an auditory system (hearing), haptic system (touch, pain), olfactory system (smell, taste) and orienting system (balance) to pick up external sensations (exteroception) and to provide internal feedback (pro-prioception). **Information**, in Gibson's sense, is contained in every aspect of sensation which is picked up by any of the body's perceptual systems (of which verbal and written material is but a small part). To the extent that this information is then used to produce appropriate reflex and voluntary responses (including further information-seeking behaviour), it can be seen to fit with the concepts of predictability and controllability outlined in the previous chapter.

Exercise

Imagine that you are sitting in an open out-patient waiting room. Think of all the sensations you might experience and what information these provide to help you make sense of what is going on around you.

One account of motion sickness, sensory conflict theory, focuses upon the internal stresses generated when information obtained via different perceptual systems is found to conflict and disrupt normal control pro-cesses. For example, the balance system may signal that the individual is moving in one direction, while the visual system signals movement in a different direction. Indeed, it is possible to induce motion sickness in a stationary individual by rotating a large drum with wavy pattern around them, which signals both rotational and up-and-down movement. In this case, conflict is generated because the eyes perceive movement, while the proprioceptive system signals that the body is stationary.

Sensory deprivation and sensory overload are both sources of loss of control and stress which can have debilitating psychological effects on individuals who are exposed to them. Sensory deprivation can lead to disorientation, chronic boredom, depression and even hallucinations.

Exercise

Think of situations in which patients are likely to be exposed to sensory deprivation and identify ways in which their monotony, lack of stimulation and/or disorientation may be relieved.

Sensory overload can lead to tension, anxiety, loss of sleep, anger and even violence. Think how you might react to neighbours who are noisy at all hours of the day and night. You might care to consider whether it is the actual noise or the lack of control over it which is important.

> **Example**
>
> Think of situations in which patients on the wards are exposed to unnecessary sensory overload. Identify simple ways in which health care professionals can reduce overload and stress for patients on the wards.

As with other areas of psychological theory, it is not necessary for health professionals to accept one theory of perception and reject the other. The two theories presented here, representational theory and direct perception, may seem entirely incompatible. However, both may usefully be applied in different circumstances. Humans are undoubtedly active seekers of information and will generally make correct interpretations when rich and accurate information is available. Thus the theory of direct perception may hold true where we have unrestricted access to all the information we need, and where the environment is relatively familiar, orderly and predictable.

The reliance upon inference, contained in representational theory, probably applies best when external information is limited, or where our access to information is restricted, or in unfamiliar, chaotic or unpredictable situations where it is difficult to make immediate sense of the information available. In these situations, the brain could be said to impose some semblance of order and predictability in order to ensure that the individual can maintain control. In fact, ambiguity and conflicting information, together with overload or restricted information, are most commonly encountered in the social – rather than the physical – environment. Hospitals are very strange social environments indeed to those who are unfamiliar with them.

> **Exercise**
>
> Next time you enter a strange situation, like a new department or placement, think about how you try to find out what is going on. Write down all the ways you gather information which will help you to know what is expected of you. How do you feel while this is happening? How do you feel afterwards and why?

Social perception

The majority of human perception takes place in a social environment in which the information available to us is shaped or constrained by the society in which we live and by those around us, whether deliberately or unintentionally. In social situations, we may actively try to seek out further information; for example, by asking other people. Alternatively, we may make the best interpretation we can on the basis of the information which is available; for example, by observing what other people are doing. When we do this, we often make mistakes. My grandfather used to tell a story of how he drove home in a thick fog in the blackout during the war, only to find that three other cars were trying to follow him into his driveway! Presumably they had all drawn inferences about where the car in front was likely to be going. Recently, a Japanese friend became lost because everyone else was going the other way and she followed them instead of the instructions she was given!

The issue of stress caused by conflicting information is particularly important in social settings. We find it difficult to know what to make of people who say one thing, but whose voice or body language signals something different. 'You'll be alright' hardly sounds reassuring when uttered by someone who looks as if things are far from alright. Likewise, we may be confused, anxious or angry when we receive different information from different people about the same thing, or when other people make a wrong diagnosis or decision because they fail to find out from us how we feel (for example, if we are in pain) or what we want (rather than what they expect us to do). The importance of non-verbal communication is considered further in Chapter 9 on social processes.

Exercise

List all the possible sources of 'information' available to an individual who is sitting in a hospital bed, or visiting an out-patient department, or being visited at home by a health care professional. Now identify all possible sources of conflicting information which may generate stress. Now consider how health professionals can help to reduce these potential areas of conflict.

Seeing things from a different viewpoint

One of the major problems which you may have encountered if you have thought seriously about the above exercise, is to imagine what it is actually like to be a patient in a hospital bed, or whatever, if this has never actually happened to you. One of the developmental tasks of childhood is to learn to take the perspective of somebody else and some famous experiments in psychology have focused upon the ability to **decentre** or be able to envisage what things look like from another viewpoint.

Piaget used a three-dimensional model of three mountains to test the ability of young children to imagine what a view would appear like from the physical position of another observer (see Gross 1992: 748). Prior to the age of about 8 years, they will choose the photograph which represents their own view, rather than that of someone situated elsewhere. These findings have been challenged by other researchers who have shown that children as young as 3 years are able to undertake less abstract tasks which involve understanding the motives and intentions of other people or characters. On the other hand, even as adults we misjudge the needs or motives of other people on occasions because we assume that they have access to the same knowledge or information that we do, or because we are unable to imagine how they are feeling. An inability to see things from the point of view of other people in certain situations is very common and is termed **egocentrism**.

Some people argue that it is not possible to know what it is like to have a baby unless we have had one ourselves, or that we cannot know what bereavement is like until we have lost someone close to us. However, health professionals are all involved with people whose experiences are well outside anything they have ever experienced themselves. The ability to imagine how people feel in such situations is called *empathy*. We may not all be able to empathize with every individual in every situation. However, we should be able to recognize that other people do not necessarily see complex situations in the same way that we do, because our different knowledge and experience of the world, together with specialized training, has shaped our perceptions.

There is now a lot of research which suggests that nurses are not very good at judging how patients feel. Several studies have showed that nurses tend to underestimate patients' feelings of pain. Johnston (1982) found that nurses were able to recognize people who were anxious, but were not very good at identifying what they were worrying about. They tended to base their observations on assumptions about what patients worry about, rather than finding out individual concerns. Patients were better at judging sources of other patients' concerns than were the nurses, perhaps because they did share similar experiences. Nurses appear to be influenced by their own cultural expectations and past experiences, and by the process of stereotyping patients, for example according to their medical diagnoses (see Chapter 9).

A simple remedy to understanding how individual patients feel and how they have interpreted what is happening to them is to undertake an individual assessment which is holistic and humanistic in the sense that it does not just focus upon medical facts about their condition, but takes into account what the patient understands about their condition, why they believe what they do, what effects their beliefs are having on their behaviour and what other concerns are influencing their perceptions. Although this may sound time-consuming, errors in communication can prove costly if they delay a patient's recovery or lead to non-compliance with important medical treatment.

Exercise

An elderly person with diabetes confided that she understood her condition was 'terminal'. Consider how this belief may have come about. How can health professionals try to ensure that this type of misapprehension does not occur?

Personal construct theory

George Kelly (see Chapters 1 and 3), a psychologist working within the humanistic tradition, was interested in how people make sense of the world around them and understand themselves in relation to others. In so doing, he proposed a unique theory called **personal construct theory**. This is normally proposed as a theory of personality, but is included here because it is primarily concerned with the way in which people learn to perceive, understand or construe themselves and their world.

Kelly invented a whole new language with which to present his theory because he did not wish it to be distorted by the use of existing terms. In so doing, he created a very sensible and useful theory which is almost totally inaccessible to the lay person in its original form. We therefore offer our own interpretation of some of the key relevant points.

Kelly envisaged all individuals as scientists in their own right. This is termed 'man-as-scientist'. According to this view, each time people are exposed to new stimuli or experiences, they form hypotheses about what is going on. They then test these to see if their predictions are correct. If they are wrong, they readjust their view or try again. This leads to the formation of **constructs**, or sets of beliefs about the world. Once a hypothesis has been tried and tested, existing beliefs or predictions are either strengthened, or challenged, or new ones formed.

Kelly proposed that all constructs are bipolar. This means that each lies on a continuum from a positive pole to a negative pole. Thus I might regard myself anywhere between dim-witted and clever, beautiful and ugly, popular and unpopular, at any particular point in time. Kelly proposed that constructs are unique to the individual (hence it is called personal construct theory). This is why, in his assessments, he allowed people to identify their own ways of describing themselves compared with others (see Chapter 1), rather than responding to a fixed set of dimensions. This is where Kelly's approach differs from methods of attitude measurement, even though some of these, such as the **semantic differential scale** and the **Likert scale**, are also bipolar. The unique method of individual assessment devised by Kelly is the **repertory grid** (see Gross 1992: 898–901). This was used to illustrate Ann's beliefs about herself in relation to others in Chapter 1, and you may wish to refer back to this before undertaking the following exercise.

Exercise

A blank repertory grid is provided in Fig. 5.1. First, identify two important people in your life (significant others) with whom you often compare yourself, and fill in their names. These may include a parent, sibling or best friend, the choice is yours. Now identify three constructs which you often use in those comparisons. For example, you may find yourself saying 'I wish I was more like C because she is so slim' or 'M is wonderful because he is so kind'. Your construct now has one pole, which may be positive or negative. For each construct, now identify the opposite pole. The opposite of kind may be unkind or cruel or vicious, depending upon how you see it, so select the opposite which suits you. When you have filled in your three positives and negatives, place a tick or a cross in each box to represent how you see yourself and your significant others.

What are the similarities and the differences between your actual self, your ideal self and your significant others? Why do you think that this is? Are your judgements realistic? (Do you think that other people make the same judgements?)

Copy out the grid, minus the tick and crosses, and give it to each of your selected significant others to fill in next time you see them. Do they see you the same as you see yourself? If there are any differences, why do you think this is? Have you learned anything about yourself?

Bipolar constructs: Positive (√) Negative (×)	Myself as I am (Actual self)	Myself as I would like to be (Ideal self)	Significant other 1:	Significant other 2:

Figure 5.1 Short form repertory grid for personal use.

Kelly also proposed that people may shuttle backwards and forwards between the positive and negative poles of their constructs as they interact with the world and gain new experiences. However, he noted that once existing constructs have been established and validated, it can become very hard to change them completely (note the similarities with aspects of persuasion in Chapter 9). Therefore, if an individual has developed the belief that they are worthless and have seen this supported by a catalogue of failures, it is very hard, subsequently, to change that belief. Kelly proposed that one of the tasks of therapy for depression was to 'loosen' these constructs, so that the individual ceases to see the world in such a fixed way. This, he suggested, could be achieved by trying out new roles and engaging with new experiences in the safety of the therapeutic environment before trying them out in the real world, as outlined in

Chapter 1. You might like to reconsider this approach in the light of Goffman's dramaturgical model which is described in Chapter 9.

Some of the concepts behind Kelly's theory are not too dissimilar to those of the cognitive–behavioural theories outlined in the previous chapter and some of the implications are somewhat similar. However, Kelly highlights the fact that it is the constructs of the patient which are of primary importance in health care, and not the constructs of the staff. Thus if health care professionals view a patient's situation and problems in terms of constructs which centre upon healing as 'curing', while the patient views healing in terms of 'caring', there is likely to be a substantial mismatch of visions, methods and goals. Kelly's theory supports the need for a client-centred approach to problem solving, with the nurse or therapist acting as facilitator.

Education, in its broadest sense, is probably one of the most important ways in which all of us continue to develop new ways of seeing the world. You may find that people you work with, or those you care for, who are less well informed or who have exposed themselves to a limited range of experiences, tend to have more rigid and often more extreme views. The study of psychology, along with sociology and the other social sciences, forces us to look at the same issues from different perspectives. In so doing, this may loosen some of our previously held assumptions and beliefs and allow us to view the world and the people in it in a much less certain and more flexible way. This can be both disconcerting and liberating. Uncertainty is the food of scientific endeavour. Using Kelly's analogy of man-as-scientist, those who are most certain about everything are least likely to learn anything new which is different from their existing view.

Exercise

We often refer to certain individuals who hold very strong and certain opinions as seeing things in 'black and white'. Think about someone you know, or have met, who falls into this category. Describe what happens when you try to argue against their beliefs. How do they respond? Why do you think this is?

Memory

Memory involves receiving, processing and encoding, storing and retrieving information. Problems may occur at any stage, although there is no evidence that information actually decays while in long-term storage. Most of the problems of forgetting occur at the time of receiving and encoding, or at the point of retrieval. In this section, these issues are explored and the implications for patient care are examined. The focus is not on memory structures, but on memory processes which have direct applications for personal use and may be applied in the context of health care.

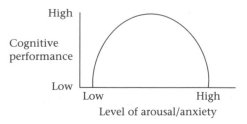

Figure 5.2 The Yerkes-Dodson law of the relationship between arousal and cognitive performance.

Attention

In order to receive any type of information, we have to pay attention to it. In other words, the information must stimulate our attention. This implies a certain state of autonomic arousal. Indeed, it has been shown that cognitive performance, including memory, is related to our level of arousal. There appears to be an inverse U relationship between arousal and cognitive performance which is termed the Yerkes-Dodson law (see Fig. 5.2). Since autonomic arousal is frequently associated with feelings of anxiety, the relationship applies equally to levels of anxiety.

A very low level of arousal reflects disinterest and inattention; therefore, memory encoding or retrieval is likely to be very poor. An extremely high level of arousal is associated with very high anxiety or even panic. In this case, the individual is likely to be distracted and unable to attend properly to any type of cognitive task; therefore, memory for information is likely to be poor, or may focus only upon the most salient aspect to them (which is not always the main point the health professional wishes to convey). The best cognitive performance is obtained from someone whose adrenaline is flowing, who is alert and slightly anxious, whose attention is focused upon the task in hand and the content of what is being said. This indicates that the patient's emotional state should be noted. Time needs to be taken to listen to and calm someone who is highly anxious, or alert someone of the importance of an issue, if they are totally unconcerned.

Two of the best places to observe the effects of high levels of arousal and anxiety are out-patient and accident and emergency departments. After instructing a patient to get up on the couch and watching him put his feet on the pillow, a colleague once observed that some people left their wits outside the door as they walked in. A more likely explanation is that the situation was very strange, frightening and confusing, and he literally could not think straight or was 'scared out of his wits'.

Even when people are attending to what is being said, their attention will tend to focus upon things which are of particular importance to them. In other words, people tend to pay attention to what they want or expect to hear and not necessarily to the things that health professionals feel are important.

Short- and long-term memory

It is generally accepted that there are two types of memory storage: short-term (**primary**) memory and long-term memory. Short-term memory is also referred to as working memory, since retention at this level is an active and conscious process. Early research using nonsense syllables and unrelated words or pictures indicated that short-term memory has a processing capacity which is limited to around seven bits of information. The combination of seven letters and digits in the British car number plate was determined by psychological research, but you will note that it is much easier to remember a number plate such as LIM1T, which effectively reduces five bits of information to one meaningful chunk, than one which reads NMG3P, which contains five unrelated bits.

The transfer of information from short- to long-term memory is facilitated by rehearsal, repetition and association. If we want to remember a telephone number, we keep repeating it until it has 'sunk in'. If we are distracted during this process, we often have to start again and look it up once more. When we are given a series of important items of information in a short space of time, there is no opportunity to rehearse any of it and this helps to explain why much of it is promptly lost.

Exercise

Next time you observe someone else give information to a patient in a clinic, write down and count how many pieces of important information they are given. Then reflect: Were they given time to repeat any of it? Did they try to do this? If you can do so, follow them outside and see how much they actually remember without prompting.

Mnemonics

Mnemonic techniques are useful ways of organizing discrete bits of information into a meaningful chunk. For example,'No Man Goes for 3p' would enhance retention of the above meaningless number plate, especially if accompanied by a visual image of a car at a toll gate. A common mnemonic for remembering the first letters of the 12 cranial nerves is: 'On Old Olympic's Towering Tops, A Fin And German Viewed Some Hops'. In the case of treatment regimens, patients could be encouraged to repeat their instructions several times and relate them to daily events (e.g. after specific meals) in order to retain the information. When trying to remember which tablet is for what, 'white for water, blue for blood, yellow for yawning (sleep)' might prove memorable if the colours of the tablets were obliging enough to conform to this mnemonic. It is probably best if patients invent their own, but they may need some encouragement. Some people prefer verbal mnemonics and others prefer visual ones. Of course, the best way we have of ensuring that we remember something is to write

it down and keep referring to it. Patients should be given written information wherever possible.

Primacy and recency effects

When people are given several pieces of information in sequence, they are
most likely to remember the thing they were told first (the **primacy
effect**) and the thing they were told last (the **recency effect**), and to
forget most of the rest. One of the reasons for this is that they have more
opportunity to mentally rehearse these items. Health professionals should
try to ensure that they give essential information first and repeat it last,
thus ensuring that the message is remembered.

Forgetting

Much forgetting is not due to the decay or loss of memories, but is
actually caused by interference when one set of memories distorts or
displaces a set of previous memories (**retroactive interference** (or inhibition)) or future memories (**proactive interference** (or inhibition)). This
may occur when patients receive differing accounts from professional and
lay sources. They eventually forget who said what and when, and become
thoroughly confused.

Have you ever had this type of experience? Someone has told you what
to do and then stressed what you should not do. All you can remember
later is the last instruction, but you cannot recall whether this is what you
should or should not do. Quite often you do it because that is all you can
remember. Perhaps this explains why patients sometimes do exactly the
opposite of what they were told to do.

Try to avoid giving patients redundant information because it can
cause interference and may lead them to do the one thing that they have
been advised *not* to do.

Mental schemas and scripts

More recent memory research has focused upon the fact that individuals
tend to encode information in relation to their own framework of understanding, which is referred to as a mental **schema** (see Chapter 3). This
allows us to organize and process large amounts of information, but it
does mean that memory encoding and recall involve a certain amount of
reconstruction. These schemas are often incorporated into a **script** by
which we construct a storyline to aid our understanding of how to behave
in particular situations, and to help in reporting sequences of events. The
map of the London underground is a good example of a schema which
was designed to help us understand the network and find our way from
A to B, even though it bears little relationship to above-ground geographi-
cal location. The script which an individual has for getting from A to B
would include details such as buying a ticket from the machine, going

down on the escalator to the Northern Line northbound, waiting for and boarding a train, changing at Oxford Circus to the Central Line, etc. The schema refers to the map; the script refers to the procedure.

It is not unusual for doctors and other health care professionals to find that a patient reports a completely different version of what happened to them, or what they were told, to the recorded account. This may be because the patient's schema is different to that of the health professional. It is therefore important to establish the patient's understanding of the situation before and after a consultation. The use of technical or medical jargon, whether spoken or written, compounds this problem, since patients will tend to make their own interpretation of something they have not fully understood.

Exercise

List the words which you use to describe medical conditions, hospital equipment or procedures, parts of the body, surgical operations or bodily functions. Now ask lay friends to define what they understand by them. You may be surprised at their lack of knowledge in comparison to your own.

Communicating effectively with patients

One of the main reasons why patients fail to follow medical advice is their inability to recall accurately what they have been told and the failure of health professionals to realize they will not remember everything. Understanding a little about memory processes can help health professionals to improve patients' recall and understanding.

The whole issue of good communication with patients and the giving of information is extremely important within the current context of health care. In fact, it is embodied in the *Patients' Charter*. Philip Ley (1988) has identified that good communication is an important component of patient satisfaction and is essential if patients are to follow medical advice. Problems of incorrect medication include not taking enough, taking too much, incorrect dose interval, incorrect treatment duration and taking additional medications, each of which can have potentially harmful consequences.

Antibiotics are among the drugs most commonly abused by the public. People frequently stop taking them once their symptoms have subsided. This can lead to the growth of resistant strains of bacteria which makes common diseases more difficult to treat. People need to be told not only the correct regimen, but understand *why* strict adherence is important to them.

The use of technical jargon is a common communication problem in health care. Words that we take for granted may be completely misinterpreted by the patient. The following delightful example was taken from the *Nursing Standard* at the time of writing:

Nurse admitting elderly lady to the ward: 'Have you ever been in-continent?'
Patient, cheerfully: 'Ooh, no dear, I can't afford it, but I have been to the Isle of Wight'.

Ley documented a catalogue of worrying research findings which demonstrate poor memory for medical information and poor understanding of medical instructions. Among the most worrying of all are findings relating to informed consent to such procedures as major surgery, chemotherapy, psychiatric review procedures, and neuroleptic drugs used in psychiatric treatment. Recall varied from about 30 per cent to about 70 per cent.

It is suggested in Chapters 4 and 6 that the term **compliance**, with its connotation of 'do what I tell you', is rather outdated in the 1990s when the current emphasis is upon patient empowerment and self-care. The philosophy of care in the National Health Service (NHS) has shifted away from one which encouraged external (powerful others) locus of control to one which encourages personal control. You may wish to bear this in mind when considering the literature on patient compliance. Doing what you are told without knowing why can sometimes lead to unfortunate and unforeseen outcomes, such as ignoring side-effects.

It has been argued that elderly people are more likely to hold external (powerful others) beliefs in control because the culture in which they grew up revered the authority of professionals such as doctors. Beisecker (1988) found that the desire for information among elderly people was as strong as that among younger people, although they were less willing to challenge medical authority. Elderly arthritis sufferers may experience painful and sometimes lethal gastrointestinal side-effects from taking anti-inflammatory drugs, even when they do not have any noticeably beneficial effect, because they are too willing to comply with repeat prescriptions, fail to associate indigestion symptoms with the tablets, and have little or no knowledge of the potential risks they are taking (Walker *et al.* 1990).

Patients rarely ask questions or say that they have not understood something because they don't want to take up valuable time and they do not wish to appear foolish. The onus is therefore on the nurse, therapist and doctor to ensure that they accurately understand what is going on. There are a number of ways in which communication between clients and health care professionals can be improved (Ley 1988), using principles from memory research:

- Improve the environment (avoid delays, be friendly, allow the patient to explain things in their own words).
- Find out what the patient believes and encourage feedback.
- Stress the importance of particular content and repeat it.
- Give important information first and repeat it last.
- Check that you are using language that the patient can understand.
- Give specific, rather than general or vague, information.
- Provide written back-up material, but ensure that this is written and presented so that people can understand it.

It is worthwhile remembering that recognition is always easier than recall. Therefore, it is better to ask an open question like 'What were you told last time?' than a closed question like 'Do you remember that last time you were told . . . ?' The patient will inevitably remember, once reminded, and will not wish to appear a fool by admitting to having forgotten.

Certain memories are context-specific and are aided by a return to the environment or emotional state in which the information was originally received (just as a certain piece of music often triggers a long forgotten event). Thus patients may have entirely forgotten what was said until returning to the sight and smell of the hospital. Only then do they remember what they should have done, but they are too embarrassed to admit that they didn't do it.

Ley claimed that effective information-giving is related to patient satisfaction as well as compliance. Support for this was found by Fleissig (1993), who demonstrated that women who had recently given birth and who felt that staff had given them enough information during labour and delivery were more likely to express satisfaction with their experience than those who wanted more information and further explanation. The important word here is 'enough'. What is sufficient for one person may be insufficient for another or information overload for a third. A colleague was recently heard to attribute her daughter's post-natal depression to an excess of choices presented to her during her pregnancy and labour. She felt that her daughter had been unable to cope with this. These observations highlight the need for individualized assessment of information needs (in other words, ask the patient if they have sufficient information, or if they would like to know more).

One situation in which it is particularly difficult to take in information is when someone is being given bad news about their condition or prognosis. Patients often fail to appreciate that bad news, for example that they have cancer, is balanced by good news about current treatment outcomes. Some health care professionals have been experimenting with tape-recording 'bad news' consultations (Fallowfield and Hogbin 1989), so that their patients can take these away to listen to them at their leisure. This, of course, would not suit everybody, but many who have elected to do this have found it extremely helpful in gaining a better understanding of the whole situation, and in explaining it to close family or friends.

Psychoanalytic explanations of forgetting

Freud argued that certain painful memories are **repressed**, or forced out of the conscious mind into the unconscious. Repression was one of a series of **defence mechanisms** he described which defend the ego, or sense of self, against harsh external realities. Another is **denial**, in which the individual fails to acknowledge the reality of a situation. These so-called unconscious psychological defences will be observed in a variety of individuals and situations. However, although they may protect against anxiety in the short term, they may lead to long-term problems through lack of acceptance. Denial can also lead to a lack of communication between the patient and those close to him or her, but it is often difficult to establish if this is a conscious or unconscious process. It is not unusual to find relatives entering into a conspiracy of silence in which everyone is suffering alone while anxiously trying to protect everyone else. Counselling, understanding and gentle guidance towards acceptance of the truth, combined with hope, may be beneficial, but it is important to beware of deciding what is best for the patient. Direct confrontation can be damaging and there are reports of patients who give up in the face of a reality they are unable to tolerate.

Not all recalled memories are necessarily accurate, as has been revealed by the controversial 'recovered memories' phenomenon. It is thought that certain childhood memories, such as those involving recollections of sexual abuse, may be repressed and only become 'remembered' in adulthood. It is not known to what extent these events are 'real' or imagined, and it is often difficult to obtain other types of evidence.

Memory loss and encoding problems

Certain types of head injury can lead to memory loss or **amnesia**. Some accidental damage causes a complete loss of short-term memory and encoding, such that the individual fails to remember anything which has occurred from a few moments ago back to the onset of the disorder or trauma. Different types of memory may be affected differently by different types of brain damage. Long-term memories for childhood autobiographical episodes or events (**episodic memory**) may be little affected, while long-term memory related to overlearned motor skills, rules or sequences (**procedural memory**) and general knowledge for facts (**semantic memory**) acquired prior to brain injury may also remain intact. Loss of memory for things which have occurred since the time of injury is probably due to failure to transfer information from the short- to the long-term store. The development of Alzheimer's disease appears to cause memory to retreat. At first, memories for the past are retained, while recent and then gradually more distant memories disappear. This can cause substantial disorientation. One of the well-known memory tests used to diagnose dementia includes asking who the current prime minister is and what day of the week it is. Confusion has already been associated with loss of control (see Chapter 4) and it is probably not surprising that dementia sufferers tend to suffer from depression (see also issues related to control, support and depression in Chapter 6).

Memory problems can make communication very difficult and take great patience and understanding. It is tempting to think that once a person's memory has gone, that the person inside has also gone. Many carers experience great distress because the person they love no longer remembers who they are, or mistakes them for a parent. People with dementia may ask the same question again and again and never appear to take in the answer. It can become very frustrating and makes the sufferer susceptible to abuse from relatives who can simply take no more. It is not easy for professionals either.

Life review in dementia

Marie Mills (see Mills and Walker 1994) conducted a series of in-depth interviews with elderly patients on a long-stay ward who had severe dementia. She encouraged them to talk about their past. She recounts how one patient, Mr Fellows, appeared initially to be very depressed. He described detailed episodes from his childhood, his school and his relationship with his parents which his wife, and his old school, confirmed as accurate. In fact, both she and the hospital staff were surprised that he was able to remember so much. He recounted how important his school cap was and how frightened he was of losing it. On reporting back to the staff, they confirmed that he would sometimes wander round the ward in an agitated state saying, 'where's my cap?'. In later interviews, Mr Fellows confided how ashamed he was of being incontinent and how annoyed he was that the chiropodist had not attended to his feet. It appeared that he was very aware of his current feelings. As the study progressed, he started to cheer up and appeared less agitated and depressed. Part of this may have been that he liked talking to the researcher (although he never remembered who she was, he appeared to associate her with something pleasant and would move towards her when she appeared on the ward). A more convincing reason might be that the staff began to respond to him differently and treated him with the respect due to an interesting character with an interesting personal history, not just an incontinent old man whose memory had gone. The importance of this is considered in more depth in Chapter 9, which looks at the relationship between stereotyping and depersonalization. Mills recommended that a detailed social history should be maintained for all long-stay patients so that staff are reminded to see the person and not just the behaviour.

It is worth remembering that simple medical conditions, such as severe anaemia, or self-neglect which can lead to malnutrition or dehydration, are common causes of mental confusion and disorientation in the elderly. Another common cause is drug **iatrogenesis** (medically induced illness). Many commonly prescribed drugs can cause confusion, especially if an overdose is taken. Non-compliance could be the cause and consequence of the problem. Correctly identifying the source of the problem and initiating appropriate treatment should reverse memory loss in these cases.

Summary

- Two alternative theories of perception (representational theory and Gibson's theory of direct perception) are presented and the circumstances in which each may apply are considered.

- The relevance of these theories to social situations is considered, with particular reference to situations where information is sparse or conflicting signals are given.

- The importance of being able to understand how things appear from the perspectives or viewpoints of others is discussed.

- Kelly's personal construct theory is outlined and its relevance to the ways that people perceive or construe the world considered.

- A number of aspects of memory research and theory are described, with particular reference to how much people remember about health advice.

- Ways of improving memory for health information are offered.

- Memory loss, its implications and relevant therapeutic approaches, are considered.

Further reading

Gross, R.D. (1992) *Psychology: The Science of Mind and Behaviour*, 2nd end. London: Hodder and Stoughton. Chapter 9.

Ley, P. (1988) *Communicating with Patients: Improving Satisfaction and Compliance*. London: Chapman and Hall.

STRESS AND COPING: THEORY AND APPLICATIONS IN HEALTH CARE

Introduction

What is stress? How do people cope with illness and adversity? Read any newspaper or magazine, watch the television, or listen to the radio and you will find the word stress. It is used both as a causal explanation, as in 'He was very stressed so he lost his job', and as an outcome, 'Losing his job made him very stressed'. The concept of stress is very confusing and lacks a clear definition. Briner (1994) has argued that stress has become a modern myth, with 'attributional power' similar to demons and witches in the Middle Ages, or 'nerves' in the 1950s. Perhaps we should abandon using the term altogether. An alternative is to think through very carefully what the concepts of stress and coping mean, and understand the various approaches that have been used.

This chapter explores three approaches to stress: the response-based definition of Selye (1956), the stimulus-based definition of Holmes and Rahe (1967) and the transactional model of Lazarus and Folkman (1984). The role of intrapersonal factors (personal beliefs and behaviours), including the Type A behaviour pattern, hardiness, self-efficacy and perceived control are considered. The ways in which interpersonal factors, such as social support, mediate stress responses are considered. These factors allow a closer look at how differences between individuals influence whether they get ill, and if they do get ill, how they cope with the experience. These concepts are related to the debate about psychological preparation for surgery, looking at the techniques that have been used and what outcome measures have been recorded. Practical advice is offered on how health care professionals can help patients cope with surgery, and how they can recognize sources of stress within their own work environment.

Theories of stress and coping

Stress has become an important topic because it is clear that the pattern of disease, especially cardiovascular disease, cannot be explained simply by physiological factors alone. Within a **biopsychosocial** model of health, it has been suggested that the complex interaction of a person's biology, psychological state and social environment determine whether they become ill or not. The exact mechanism of these interactions remains unclear, although it is thought that one of the factors may be the way the immune system functions. A new research area called **psychoneuro-immunology** studies the way that the thoughts and feelings a person has can influence the way their brain functions and how the immune system responds. A fully functioning immune system is needed to prevent infections and certain types of cancer from developing. The development of AIDS in people with HIV provides a good example of this. There is already some evidence that after very stressful events like bereavement, levels of immune functioning are reduced (Schulz and Schulz 1992). At this stage, it is not possible to determine precisely how the mind, social world and body interact to result in illness for some people but not others. Much more research is required before this process is fully understood. In the meantime, it is necessary to assess the relevance of theoretical models of stress.

A response-based model of stress

It is common to attribute the introduction of the concept of stress to Hans Selye, although Cannon first wrote about the 'fight or flight response' in the early part of this century. The **fight or flight response** occurs when a person is in an emergency situation which is perceived to be very threatening. This response is a physiological one in which arousal of the sympathetic nervous system results in release of adrenaline and noradrenaline. These chemical neurotransmitters activate the body by causing the release of glucose stored in the liver (needed for muscular activity), increasing cardiovascular activity by increasing the heart rate and blood pressure, increasing the viscosity of the blood, re-routing of blood from the digestive organs and skin to the brain and muscles, increasing the rate and depth of breathing and widening the pupils of the eyes. Cannon suggested that this state of arousal temporarily disrupts **homeostasis** (the normal state of physiological balance) until successful action to deal with the threat allows a return to a stable state.

The reason this response is termed 'fight or flight' was based upon observations that the most common animal responses to threat from other animals involves fighting them or running away. It was presumed that these responses evolved over the history of human beings because they were adaptive. They prepared people to fight to retain their territory (unfortunately this included fighting each other) and enabled people to escape from dangerous situations. Modern technology has rather altered these situations, so fighting may be done by long-range weapons and 'running away' may be by car. This has been taken to imply that these physiological responses may now be rather maladaptive. It has been argued that prolonged or repeated arousal with no opportunity to engage in physical activity might actually give rise to health problems, such as hypertension. However, even when physical action is not appropriate to deal with today's problems, autonomic arousal is still necessary to prompt problem-solving activities and energize more appropriate coping actions. Therefore, Cannon's work is still relevant to underpin our understanding of the stress response.

Selye developed these ideas into a theoretical model of stress called the general adaptation syndrome (GAS), which is shown in Fig. 6.1. Selye (1956) described stress as a 'non-specific response to any demand made upon the body'. He proposed that different types of stimuli such as toxins, heat or cold, would result in a similar physiological response resulting from the release of corticosteroids. He later added psychological stressors to his list of stressful stimuli.

The GAS has three phases. It is hypothesized that the body has a normal level of resistance to stress (shown as the horizontal line in Fig. 6.1). In Phase 1, the initial alarm reaction results in a slight reduction in resistance to stress (*shock*), which then reverts to an above normal level in the *countershock* phase. In the second phase, *resistance* remains high until the final stage of *exhaustion*, where resistance rapidly drops. Phase 3, which is described as *collapse*, results in the appearance of disease or ultimately death.

Selye's account of stress was based upon animal experimentation and explained a number of important physiological processes. It has been very influential in understanding the development of stress-related illnesses, but it fails to explain individual differences in the development of these. Some people appear to lead very demanding stressful lives, but not all become ill. Furthermore, Mason (1971) has produced evidence that different stimuli result in specific responses. This challenges Selye's suggestion that

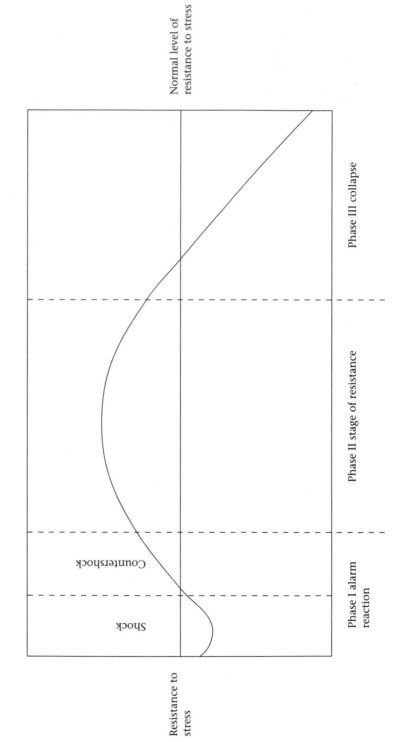

Figure 6.1 The general adaptation syndrome (adapted from Cox 1978).

there is a single stress response. The GAS is a useful model for explaining physiological processes which may lead to stress-related illnesses. Although it tells us little about the psychological components of stress, it highlights the need to consider needs for physiological homeostasis alongside psychological processes.

Exercise

Ranjan is 57 years old. He works hard managing his own fruit retail business. He enjoys playing cricket and going camping with his family. He has just had an accident at home which results in severe burns to his right arm and back. Using Selye's GAS model, predict what Ranjan's immediate responses to his accident will be. What sort of biological, psychological and social factors threaten Ranjan's long-term return to health? What might you do, as a health professional, to help Ranjan return to his normal state of health?

A stimulus-based model of stress

An alternative approach to understanding stress is to focus on the stimuli (called **stressors**) which provoke a stress reaction. In this approach, there is no assumption that all stress responses are equally important. Holmes and Rahe proposed that life changes or **life events**, either positive or negative, are stressors which tax the adaptational capacity of people, causing physical and psychological strain. They hypothesized that this strain resulted in a greater likelihood of developing health problems, including physical illness, anxiety and depression.

Holmes and Rahe (1967) investigated their theory by developing the popular social readjustment rating scale (SRRS). They identified a list of 43 common events that might happen to people and gave marriage the arbitrary score of 50. People were asked to rank order all the other events. Loss of a spouse was perceived to be the most stressful and this was given the arbitrary total of 100. All events were given scores, including events that are assumed to be pleasurable, such as going on holiday or Christmas festivities. A selection of these events is given in Table 6.1.

The researchers were not concerned with whether the event could be construed as positive or negative, but they thought that all changes required people to make some adaptations in their life. It was the change that they assumed was stressful and could influence physical health. In research using the SRRS, people are asked to tick off each event they have experienced over a set period, usually 1–2 years. The scores are then added up (called life-change units) to provide a total for each person. It is hypothesized that people with higher scores of life-change units are more likely to experience physical and/or mental illness. There is some evidence for this, but generally the correlation (a statistical measure of association) between occurrence of life events and subsequent illness is fairly low, which suggests that there are other factors involved.

Table 6.1 Measuring life stress: The life-change scale (adapted from Holmes and Rahe 1967).

Life event	Life-change unit
Death of spouse	100
Divorce	73
Marital separation	65
Jail term	63
Death of close family member	63
Personal injury	53
Marriage	50
Fired from job	47
Marital reconciliation	45
Retirement	45
Pregnancy	40
Change in eating habits	15
Vacation	13
Christmas	12
Minor violations of the law	11

Exercise

The SRRS was developed over 25 years ago. It is possible that changes in society have resulted in new or different stressors. Can you identify important life events which are causing a lot of distress in the 1990s? List the major life changes that have happened to you in the last 2 years. Compare these with a friend and see how they differ.

An important criticism of the SRRS is that it does not account for individual appraisals of the meaning of various life events. For example, a divorce may be a very welcome relief from a disruptive, conflict-filled marriage, or result from a painful betrayal of trust in an otherwise happy relationship. Some important life events can give rise to ambiguous perceptions. For example, childbirth may bring a baby that is very much wanted, but the mother may, at the same time, regret her loss of freedom. The wording of the SRRS is rather vague and 'Change in health of family member' may refer to a terminal illness or a relatively minor problem. Once again, it is likely that illness in the family has a differential impact on people. Some people cope well with a major problem, while others appear to fall apart as the result of a relatively trivial one. The total score of the SRRS can result from many different stressors, so in a practical way it does little to tell us how to help people. It simply highlights them as being potentially vulnerable to physical or mental illness.

A particular controversy remains in the aetiological significance of stressful life events for cancer, despite much research in the area. One problem is that it is very uncertain how long cancers develop in the body before they can be recognized. Most life-events research asks people to recall events over the last couple of years, but it is possible that some cancers may be present for many years before they are discovered. If people are asked to remember back over many months or even years, there may be some distortion in their memories with either very good or very bad events being forgotten. Another problem is that, if we ask people who are diagnosed with cancer to recall life events, their memories may be biased. In retrospect, certain events may appear more salient *because* they subsequently developed cancer. Chapter 2 referred to this in describing how people actively search for explanations of disease.

Daily hassles

A final problem with the stimulus approach is the emphasis on major stressors or life events. In everyday life, major life changes like bereavement, divorce or imprisonment, thankfully occur relatively infrequently, yet people report that they experience stress and also develop diseases. Perhaps it is a cumulation of the minor annoying things like missing the bus, being late for work or spilling the coffee, which determine the probability of becoming ill.

Lazarus and his colleagues (see Kanner *et al.* 1981) proposed that the presence of negative experiences (**daily hassles**) and positive experiences (*daily uplifts*) could influence health. There is some evidence that daily hassles may be associated with health outcomes, although it is unclear if it is the quantity of hassles experienced or their personal meaning that causes changes to health. However, there is less support for the notion that experiencing 'uplifts' can somehow buffer the effects of stress. This is a comparatively new area of research and there is much that is not yet known.

Exercise

The following 12 hassles are taken from a Daily Hassles Index for College Students in America (Schafer 1992):

- parking problems
- library too noisy
- too little time
- too little money
- doing the laundry
- deciding what to wear
- books unavailable in the library
- getting up in the morning
- my weight
- noisy neighbours
- boring teacher
- constant pressures of studying

Rate yourself over the last 2 days. What other hassles did you experience? Ask a client or patient in your current clinical placement about their daily hassles and list these. Now compare the two lists. How many are similar? Why are there differences? What can health professionals do to reduce daily hassles for their clients/patients?

A transactional model of stress and coping

Stimulus-based models of stress, like response-based models, have their origins in an engineering conceptualization. People are assumed to show the effects of certain levels of strain in the way that mechanical structures, like bridges, do. Is this a reasonable way to understand people? Perhaps one of the major differences between bridges and people is that people have the capacity to think. Thinking can, of course, make stress either better or worse. This is why the cognitive model of stress, presented below, is particularly important.

Richard Lazarus developed an interactional theory of stress, which is shown in Fig. 6.2. According to Lazarus and Folkman (1984), 'stress is a particular relationship between the person and the environment that is appraised by the person as taxing or exceeding his or her resources and endangering his or her well-being'. Central to this theory is an assumption that anything is potentially stressful. The degree to which an event is threatening is a feature of the **cognitive appraisal** (evaluation made in the person's mind) of a specific individual. Individuals may appraise an event, such as a fall down stairs, in different ways depending upon the context. For instance, a fall down stairs which results in no obvious injury for a fit young woman may be regarded as a trivial matter (even causing some hilarity), but if the same woman was pregnant or disabled, the appraisal of threat might be very different.

According to Lazarus and Folkman (1984), people engage in a two-stage process of appraisal (see Fig. 6.2). **Primary appraisal** determines whether the event represents a threat to that individual. There are three possible outcomes to the initial appraisal: the event may be disregarded as irrelevant; it may be evaluated as a positive event which enhances well-being; or it may be seen to be a potential **threat** to well-being. If the latter appraisal is made, the individual moves to a **secondary appraisal** process. In this the individual assesses their coping resources. These include a range of environmental factors such as tangible things like money or services, or the availability of social support or help, or the knowledge and skills which enable the individual to take direct personal action to reduce or eliminate the threat.

The ways that individuals cope with potentially threatening situations also depend upon their **coping style** (the relatively stable ways in which individuals usually deal with difficult situations). In addition, people take account of what else is happening in their life, both good and bad. The outcome of this complex appraisal process is likely to be the coping responses or **coping strategies** that people use to deal with the threat.

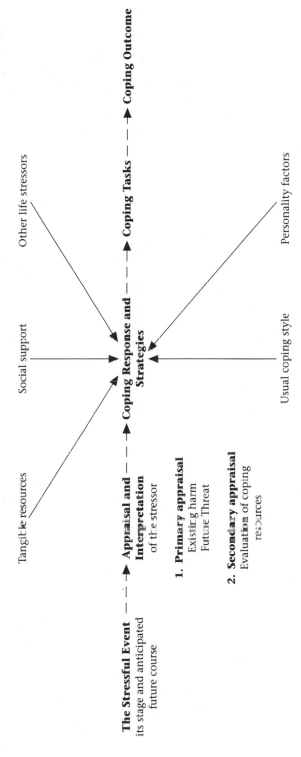

Figure 6.2 Transactional model of stress (adapted from Lazarus and Folkman 1984).

Lazarus and Folkman suggest that coping responses may either be emotion-focused or problem-focused. In **emotion-focused coping**, the objective is to reduce the feeling of distress or fear associated with the threat. You might note the influence of psychoanalysis here. For example, an individual may choose to deny the existence of the threat, which could allow them to continue with their everyday life by re-appraising the situation as non-threatening. An alternative response is called **problem-focused coping**, in which the individual actively seeks ways to mitigate or deal with the threat. It has been proposed that problem-focused coping results in a better outcome because the threat is dealt with. However, emotion-focused coping may be adaptive at certain stages, as it might help to reduce anxiety to a level where people are able to consider their options more calmly. Other researchers have classified coping into **active** or **passive coping strategies**, which imply doing something versus doing nothing or relying upon others (Rosenstiel and Keefe 1983); or **approach** (confronting reality and dealing with problems) versus **avoidance** (see Miller 1992). You may note the similarities between these classifications. Further consideration is given to their effectiveness in Chapter 8 in the section on chronic pain.

Successful coping is usually referred to as **adaptation** or adjustment, while unsuccessful coping is usually referred to as **maladaptation**. One of the problems with these definitions is that it can vary depending upon whose perspective you take. Relying on others may be regarded as adaptive from the point of view of an individual who receives care, but maladaptive from the point of view of those upon whom they are dependent. Doing nothing is adaptive if the situation is best left alone, but may be fatal if direct action is required. Some maladaptive coping strategies involve the use of substances, such as alcohol, cigarettes and illegal drugs, which dull the senses and provide an illusion of well-being. They are classified as maladaptive because they not only fail to deal with the problems the individual has, but can actually make them worse by creating additional financial, personal or health problems. This means that a coping strategy can become an additional stressor.

The Lazarus theory conceptualizes stress and coping as a reciprocal and dynamic process in which all factors are regarded as mutually causative. Thus people receive feedback from their appraisals of their own coping attempts which influences how situations are perceived.

Case Study: Lisa

Lisa is a 16-year-old girl who is 36 weeks pregnant. She has just been told by her parents that she cannot return to their home once she has had her baby. Lisa will think about how this will affect her (primary appraisal). She could decide that it is irrelevant, as she has already got a flat with her 21-year-old partner. She could decide that it is a good thing that her parents have asked her not to return to their home, because she has been trying to pluck up the courage to tell them that she is moving in with her partner after the birth. Thus their message has increased her feeling of well-being and prevented any arguments. Alternatively, Lisa could regard this as a threat because she has nowhere else to go. If this is the case, Lisa will have to consider her options (secondary appraisal). What resources does she have to cope with this threat? She might have a rich grandmother who has just died leaving her lots of money to buy a flat (tangible resources). Or she might have a married sister who is willing to take her in and provide her with help in caring for the baby (social support). How does Lisa usually cope when things go wrong (coping style)? Does Lisa normally cope with situations herself, or does she just hope for something to turn up, or will she rely on others to sort it out (active or passive coping strategies)? What else is happening in Lisa's life at the moment (concurrent life stress)? Is Lisa struggling to overcome a drug-taking habit? Is Lisa in the middle of GCSE examinations? What is the effect on Lisa? Could it influence her to go into premature labour? Is she anxious about her problems? Has she become depressed?

Exercise

Using a transactional model of stress and coping, and the story of Lisa, how can health professionals intervene to enhance her coping outcome? List all the actions that you think might be helpful for Lisa. Can you think of any actions which might make Lisa's situation worse? Why?

Lazarus and Folkman's model has become very popular, as it clearly addresses the psychological and behavioural components of coping. It has been adapted to a nursing context by Benner and Wrubel (1989), who provide a detailed analysis of the relationship between stress, coping and caring in different contexts. However, there are a number of criticisms. First, this model fails to adequately account for physiological processes. Second, it is very much an individual model which suggests that people have a range of possible coping responses open to them. This might not be the case, for example, in families where the range of possible coping responses for a mother of young children may be quite restricted. It may also be insufficient for understanding complexities in family coping, such as when the mother has a chronic illness (see Stetz *et al.* 1986). Finally, there is an assumption that cognitive appraisals actually take place, although there is very little evidence to support this. People commonly respond to everyday events out of habit or convention. It may be that only major events are sufficiently salient to trigger the degree of cognitive processing proposed by the Lazarus model. There is also the possibility that people who are flexible in using different types of response to deal with different types of situation may cope better with stress overall (see Cohen and Edwards 1989).

Psychological adjustment: Anxiety and depression

When coping outcomes are positive, such as passing an exam, we usually feel pleased and experience an increase in our self-confidence. What seemed stressful at the time may be evaluated later as a challenge. The psychological consequences of negative outcomes include **anxiety** and **depression**. Both of these are normal responses to stressful situations but can have serious disabling effects when they are experienced as intense and/or chronic conditions. The issue of mental illness is beyond the remit of this book. However, anxiety and depression as normal responses to stress are considered below. The boundary between what is normal and what is not is clearly a contentious issue. Help-seeking is often determined by individuals who can no longer cope with their feelings, or by health professionals who find it difficult to help individuals to cope with their feelings, or by relatives, friends or carers who find that the individual's behaviour is having a detrimental effect on themselves or those around them. If in doubt, it is probably wise to seek the advice of a doctor who may wish to refer to a clinical psychologist, psychiatrist, mental health nurse or social worker, depending upon the type of problem.

Mild anxiety was examined from a number of theoretical perspectives in Chapter 1. It is associated with autonomic arousal which accompanies the alarm or 'fight or flight' responses to perceived threat identified above. This is normally quickly resolved as the individual assesses their coping resources and implements effective coping strategies to reduce or eliminate the threat. For example, when I find myself on a collision course with someone else, I step quickly out of the way. However, there are situations in which primary and secondary appraisal fail to identify an appropriate course of action. These are summed up as follows:

- Uncertainty: 'I don't know what is going
                      on'   (primary appraisal)
- Unpredictability: 'I don't know that is going
                      to happen'   (primary appraisal)
- Uncontrollability: 'I don't know what I can
                      do about it'   (secondary appraisal)
                      'There is nothing I can do
                      about it'   (secondary appraisal)
                      'There is nothing anyone
                      can do about it'   (secondary appraisal)

Perceived uncertainty and unpredictability are associated with anxiety. Perceived uncontrollability (hopelessness) is associated with depression. Remember that individual perceptions are based upon personal experiences and are therefore likely to vary. Some individuals who are depressed or anxious may actually be in situations which are beyond their control, while others have had negative past experiences so that they cannot see any way of gaining control over even a simple situation (see Seligman's learned helplessness model in Chapter 4).

Uncertainty, unpredictability and uncontrollability may be inherent in the situation. Sudden bereavement is an example of a totally unpredictable and uncontrollable event. Many daily hassles involve sudden or unpredictable events, like falling over. Social factors, such as unemployment or poverty, may (or may not) be beyond the control of the individual. On the other hand, uncertainty and unpredictability may reflect lack of information, knowledge or education on the part of the individual. This is why information-giving and patient education are important anxiety-reducing components of hospital treatment and care. Uncontrollability may reflect lack of practical or social skills, or tangible resources, which would enable an individual to deal successfully with the situation. Therefore, teaching patients breathing and relaxation exercises and providing a handy alarm bell all contribute to stress reduction in hospital care. Above all, health professionals need to avoid giving conflicting information, since this ensures lack of control.

Depression due to perceived uncontrollability may be due to one major uncontrollable event, as in post-traumatic stress, or to repeated experiences of loss of control over a long period. A history of childhood abuse may predispose someone to depression because of a deep sense of loss of control and long-term damage to self-confidence and self-esteem. Much minor depression is self-limiting because, as circumstances change or knowledge is gained, control improves.

Psychological treatments for depression may utilize any of the models outlined in Chapter 1. Clinical depression often includes self-neglect and intentions to self-harm and therefore may require the temporary removal of the individual to a safe hospital environment. A cognitive–behavioural approach would analyse the current situation and seek to identify achievable short term goals, together with the coping skills necessary to achieve them. New skills (e.g. social skills) are taught and the individual learns that it is possible to achieve successful outcomes. They would, at the same time, learn to recognize unrealistic negative thoughts and replace them with realistic positive ones. A plan of action would guide them towards the successful accomplishment of longer-term goals. These approaches have been demonstrated to be successful and are recommended as an adjunct to anti-depressants, so that the individual will learn effective coping skills to prevent future relapse. However, it should be remembered that attributing depression solely to individual psychological or physiological factors, rather than situational factors, may be an example of the **fundamental attribution error** (see Chapter 9). A full analysis of external factors, such as personal relationships, work environment and sociopolitical factors, should be taken into account and addressed (see the summary in Table 6.2 at the end of this chapter).

Coping with medical procedures

Undergoing a medical procedure, whether an investigation or treatment, is potentially a very stressful experience. Even apparently minor (to health professionals) procedures, such as having a chest X-ray, can cause anxiety because of the uncertainty involved.

Exercise

List all of the uncertainties you can think of which could be involved in attending for a chest X-ray. How many of these could be reduced or eliminated by providing patients with adequate information?

Being admitted to hospital is usually perceived to be a major disruption to an individual's lifestyle. Common complaints are a lack of independence, lack of privacy, boredom, loss of control and the sense of depersonalization which occurs with the role change to a 'patient'. It has been suggested that frequent causes of anxiety and stress prior to surgery include: fear of the unknown; worries about the disease; worries about surgery, especially about the anaesthetic and the possibility of altered body image or mutilation; worries about families; and worries about employment and financial matters.

To address these concerns, it has been recommended that patients are psychologically prepared prior to surgery. The rationale for preparation has been based on a number of commonsense and theoretical assumptions. In the current ethos of consumer rights and the *Patients' Charter*, it is assumed that people have a right to know what will happen to them, and further that such knowledge reduces anxiety. From a theoretical perspective, it may be seen from other parts of this book that concepts like perceived control, learned helplessness, pain management and cognitive appraisal could modify the experience of stress. Many different methods of preparation for surgery have been tried. All of these are based upon psychological theories which have been explored in this book.

- *Procedural information* – the order in which events will happen.
- *Sensory information* – how the patient is likely to feel.
- *Behavioural information* – how the patient should act at each stage.
- *Relaxation training* – how to reduce muscular tension using exercises and breathing.
- *Teaching cognitive and behavioural coping responses* – teaching or modelling how to use 'positive' self talk or active coping behaviours which deal effectively with the problem.

These techniques have been delivered to patients in a variety of ways, including one-to-one sessions with a nurse or therapist, group sessions, by showing a video or in a leaflet. A patient who is adequately prepared may experience the following benefits:

- A reduction in anxiety and distress.
- A reduction in the experience of pain.
- A reduction in the use of analgesics (but note that this is not necessarily the same as experiencing less pain).
- A shorter hospital stay.
- Increased mobility.
- Faster clinical recovery, such as better wound-healing and less infection.

The hospital as an institution may also experience benefits, including:

- Shorter hospital stays means more patients can be treated.
- Reductions in analgesic use means lower drugs expenditure.
- A reduction in costs.

There have been many research studies to evaluate the effectiveness of psychological preparation (e.g. Hayward 1975). Overall, they demonstrate that most methods are effective but there is insufficient evidence to know which is the best method for a particular patient. A more serious criticism is that in attempting to alter the responses of individual patients, we are ignoring the conditions within hospitals which are engendering stress (Hallett 1991). Thus by labelling patients as 'anxious' and providing 'anxiety-reducing information', we place on them the responsibility to change their responses without considering structural factors within the organization of hospitals, such as the inflexible ways in which care is delivered. It may be that hospital services need modification, rather than the patients who use them. A patient-centred approach is essential to ensure that the individual has as much or as little information as they can cope with. Information overload can be as dangerous as information deficit and the best way to determine individual needs is through a process of individual negotiation (ask the patient!). Some patients will say, 'Don't tell me – you just get on with it'.

FOCUS ON RESEARCH

Preparing children for day surgery

Many children (as well as adults) now undergo surgery as day patients. Day-case surgery is thought to reduce the adverse effects of hospitalization for young children and has financial advantages for the institution. Ellerton and Merriam (1994) described a research study that evaluated a preparation programme for children aged 3–15 years undergoing planned surgery in Canada. The Saturday before surgery, each child and their family were invited to a group session at the Day Surgery Unit. They were shown a video which demonstrated coping behaviours, and then the child was introduced to routine pre-operative procedures like having their temperature taken. The child was taken on a tour of the operating area where they rehearsed events like saying 'good-bye' to their parents. The parents were then seen separately by a nurse who explained about post-operative side-effects and their role in caring for their child. During this time, the child was allowed to play with dolls and hospital equipment. The researchers found that fewer children and parents who had attended the programme reported high anxiety levels immediately before surgery. However, the measures were taken retrospectively, just before discharge, so might be biased by memory recall errors. Interestingly, those parents and children who had had previous surgery were more anxious than those who had none.

Exercise

What types of information were provided for (1) the children and (2) the parents? What differences in the programme would you make for 3-, 8- and 15-year-old children and their families? How would you evaluate the effectiveness of these programmes?

Social support

People are essentially social. We live in families and within communities. We form relationships with other people and the context of a person's life is populated with relatives, friends, colleagues and strangers. People are described in relation to the presence or absence of others; as being un-married, married, or having children. Relationships are the focus of this section, which will examine how the support derived from social relation-ships might help people cope with stress, and how this influences health outcomes.

Exercise

Consider your own interpersonal relationships and complete these sentences.
I am . . .
I live with . . .
I work/study with . . .

You may have described yourself as a wife, husband, mother or father. We often define ourselves in relation to others. These definitions specify the social roles which we are expected to perform. For example, being a mother implies that one has to care for children. You may live in a family, with a partner, or share a flat with friends. We often feel sorry for people who are alone and most of us fear loneliness. Most people work or study with others and work or study colleagues are often important sources of social support. They help each other to cope with daily hassles by shared understanding, acceptance and validation. Nursing students often form close mutually reinforcing ties with each other. These ties may contribute to feelings of success and the prevention of **burnout**, which refers to a type of work-related stress which is specific to the caring professions and interferes with the ability to care for others (see Taylor 1991).

This section starts by differentiating between social support and social networks and will examine various types of support. It is apparent from the research that not all support is perceived as appropriate or helpful.

Health psychologists have investigated social support because it may alter the effects of stress and prevent or reduce the effects of illness. Cobb (1976) defined social support as 'information leading individuals to believe they are cared for and loved, esteemed and valued, and belong to a network of communication and mutual obligation'. Researchers have become interested in how interpersonal relationships may protect people from the undesirable consequences of stress. Perhaps the knowledge that someone cares for you, that what you say and do are important, and that you are included in social activities helps you to cope with stress. However, as most of us know, living within a family, or with a partner, can be demanding as well as supportive. People have conflicts, they argue and criticize.

Social support is first encountered by children in the relationships they form with their parents or carers in early life. According to Bowlby (1969), successful child-rearing requires strong bonds of love to develop between the mother and child (see Chapter 7). Children who have these stable attachments are better able to learn and grow up into healthy adults. In addition, these early relationships may provide a template or model which enables the development of subsequent relationships.

Early research measures were concerned with the availability of social support. People were asked about other members of their household, and whether they had neighbours and relatives living nearby. However, just knowing that certain people were available was not enough. People may be available but non-supportive. Certain sources of support are perceived to be more credible and acceptable. For example, advice about a disease may be regarded as useful from a doctor but not from a neighbour. More recently, researchers have been concerned about the perception of availability and appropriateness of specific aspects of social support. For example, an elderly man may have kindly neighbours, but if they work all day they cannot take him a cooked meal at midday. Indeed, he may not want them to bring him food because he may regard it as charity or an invasion of privacy. He may prefer to receive 'Meals-on-Wheels', which he pays for. Thus help from other people may only be perceived as supportive in certain circumstances. It is not the act itself but the individual's perception of the meaning of the act that renders it supportive. For a review of research on the relationship between social support and health, see Callaghan and Morrissey (1993).

Exercise

What kinds of social support might someone who has just had a baby expect to receive from (1) their partner, (2) their mother, (3) their midwife and (4) their neighbour?

Social network

A social network is a system of social ties, such as those formed between family, relatives and friends. Some people develop, or are born with, lots of social ties in a community. Perhaps you can think of a person who is a member of a large extended family, most of whose members live in the same village or town. Other people are more socially isolated, maybe because they are elderly and many of their family and friends have died, or perhaps because they have recently moved to a new town or country. Of course, modern communications (e.g. the telephone) means that geographically spread people can still maintain close contact if they wish. With current health care trends, more people are receiving some or all of their care in the community. This has implications for how nurses assess and utilize social networks (for a review in mental health nursing, see Simmons 1994).

Social networks are defined in terms of their *structural properties*:

- *Size* – the number of people within the network.
- *Network density* – the amount of contact between members.
- *Accessibility* – the ease with which members can be contacted. Is it a matter of walking down the street or flying half way around the world?
- *Stability over time* – the duration the relationships have survived.
- *Reciprocity* – the amount of give and take in the relationships. People generally feel more comfortable in relationships which are built on equal amounts of give and take. Yet some relationships are very unequal in this regard, perhaps because one member is of unequal social status.
- *Content* – the nature of the involvement in the relationships (e.g. members of the same club or school class).
- *Intensity* – the degree of closeness within the relationships.

Exercise

Think about the reciprocity in the following relationships. How equal are they likely to be and why?

- nurse–patient
- grandmother–grandchild
- boss–worker
- student–teacher
- husband–wife

Berkman (see Simmons 1994) suggested that there are seven functions of a social network:

1 *Intimacy* – to enable people to express their feelings freely.
2 *Social integration* – opportunities to share experiences and ideas.
3 *Nurturing others* – opportunities to care for others.
4 *Reassurance of worth* – to provide feedback which enhances self-esteem.
5 *Assistance* – the direct exchange of goods and services with others.

6 *Guidance and advice* – feedback from others.

7 *Access to new contacts* – meeting new people or ideas.

Types of social support

There are a number of different types of support which have been identified. Each acts in a different way. Some involve 'doing for', some encourage personal action, while others involve just 'being there'.

Informational support refers to the provision of knowledge relevant to the situation the individual is experiencing. The advice given by a grandmother to a new mother about child care is an example of this type of support. A person can draw on the experiences of others as support or guidance in their own life. Just knowing that others have experienced the same life changes can be felt as supportive. This is the basis for sharing of experiences in self-help groups. Doctors and nurses can also provide informational support when, for example, they describe the possible side-effects of a treatment.

Tangible support refers to specific activities that others provide which are perceived to be helpful. For example, this may be assistance with housework or child care for a mother with a new baby. Perhaps a friend may drive a patient to a clinic appointment, or people may give money to enable a person to have special medical treatment.

Emotional support is the perceived availability of thoughtful, caring individuals who can share thoughts and feelings. Many people develop intimate relationships in which they feel safe and loved. Men seem to derive most support from their wives, while women may also form intimate confiding relationships with other women. The presence of these emotionally supportive relationships appears to be particularly important in the maintenance of mental health.

Affirmation or validatory support is given when others acknowledge the appropriateness of a person's beliefs and feelings. It prevents a person from feeling odd or strange. It suggests a sharing of feelings and prevents isolation. Nurses may be able to help patients realize that they are not alone in feeling frightened the night before an operation. Nurses can reflect back to patients that feeling angry, sad or happy may all be appropriate emotions at various periods during recovery from surgery. The encouragement of open expression of beliefs and feelings can function as a form of social support.

Social affiliation refers to one's system of mutual obligations and reciprocal help with other individuals and institutions. This is very similar to a social network. People provide services for each other from which they all derive benefits, such as a babysitting group. Obligations are based upon previous services. Many people may wish to care for their elderly parents because of the care they received as children, and their emotional attachments.

Hobfoll (1988) suggested that people with close social networks have people around them who recognize when they are under stress, off colour or poorly and persuade them to report it to a doctor, or take a holiday, or take another appropriate form of coping action. He suggested that those with poor social skills are less subject to this form of 'social prodding' because they lack a social network.

Exercise

The following are questions about social support adapted from Sarason *et al.* (1990). You may like to answer them. Think about what type of support they refer to.

1 Whom can you really count on to listen to you when you need to talk?
2 Whom can you really count on to be dependable when you need help?
3 With whom can you totally be yourself?
4 Who do you think really appreciates you as a person?
5 Whom can you count on to console you when you are very upset?

How does social support work?

Little is known about the underlying processes through which social support may affect health outcomes, but the following are some possible mechanisms.

1 Social support may influence whether a person comes into contact with possible disease-causing factors. For instance, a person in a stable sexual relationship is less likely to be exposed to sexually transmitted diseases than those who have many sexual partners.
2 Social support may influence whether a person falls ill easily or not. For example, recently widowed people experience more illness than married women of the same age.
3 Social support may affect the behaviours that people perform which prevents them from becoming ill. For example, elderly people who live alone are less likely to eat nourishing food than those who are married.
4 Social support may help people to seek medical services promptly once they have a disease. Women who discover a breast lump commonly turn to a female relative, such as a sister, for advice. If this person knows that a breast lump might be a sign of breast cancer, they can encourage the woman to seek medical help without delay.
5 Social support may modify the severity of the disease or the outcome of the disease, or life event. Women with less support are more likely to experience problems during their pregnancy (Oakley 1992).

Not all social support is helpful. Ross and Mirowsky (1989) identified from survey data that people who regularly use talking to others as a strategy for coping with stressful situations tended to be more depressed.

In addition, there is evidence from the literature on chronic pain (e.g. Flor *et al.* 1987) that those with more solicitous spouses tend to have more pain and be more depressed (see also Chapter 8). This suggests that the 'doing for' type of support is not adaptive either. The best type of social support appears to be that which raises self-esteem and self-efficacy, which probably means supporting people to help themselves.

Exercise

Think about a person you have recently cared for or helped, and describe the types of support you were able to offer. How acceptable were these and how effective do you think they were?

The balance of control and support

The theoretical relationship between perceived control, perceived support and psychological distress is illustrated in Fig. 6.3. This uses the example of someone requiring care. It could equally be applied in situations of illness, disability, unemployment or poverty. The two axes represent

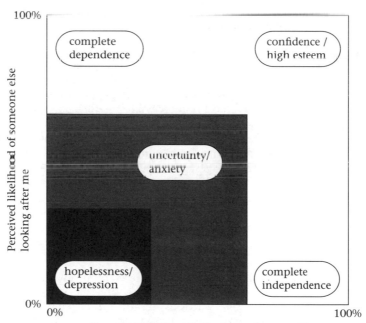

Figure 6.3 The relationship between perceived personal control, perceived support, confidence, anxiety and depression (from Walker 1989).

perceived personal control and perceived support, expressed in terms of percentage probability. It should be noted that these are based upon perceptions. Perceptions usually reflect the reality of experience, but where they deviate temporarily or permanently, it is the perceptions of control and support which appear to determine emotional response.

The best position to be in, according to both theory and research, is to have personal control over a situation, while having the assurance of available support if required. Relying solely upon other people is never the best long-term option. Paid carers may have other demands on their time, or go home from their shift, or may change their job. Even devoted carers may become ill (informal carers often suffer from stress-related illness) or may die unexpectedly. Empowerment, therefore, involves enabling people to maximize their level of personal control, while ensuring that they feel they have adequate support.

Exercise

Imagine you are ill in a hospital bed. You want a bed pan and ring the bell. How likely is it that your demand will be met immediately? If you have to wait, what will you think and how will you feel? How long are you likely to wait before you try to get out to the toilet on your own?

FOCUS ON

RESEARCH

Personal control versus social support

Ross and Mirowsky (1989) conducted a large-scale survey which they used to examine the relationships between self-report of personal control and support, coping strategies and depression. They found that people who had a high score on personal control had a low depression score and gained no additional benefit from social support in terms of positive mood. Those who scored high on social support also had a low depression score and gained no additional benefit from personal control. Their data are congruent with the theoretical model given in Fig. 6.3. This suggests that personal control and social support substitute for each other in order to protect individual well-being.

Interference and anger

One person's enthusiastic desire to help can be interpreted by another as interference, particularly if the individual wishes to be able to deal with things themselves. In this situation, interference can generate annoyance and even anger. Anger and violent outbursts are often overlooked as responses to stress caused by loss of control. They may be prompted in hospital by what is perceived by the patient to be a violation of their privacy or autonomy, or the deliberate removal of personal control, particularly when the individual has no appropriate means of dealing with the situation themselves. This is particularly likely in patients who are already in a state of fear, anxiety or confusion. A typical example is that of an elderly or confused person who is admitted to a strange hospital or nursing home environment and who is then expected to conform to the routines of getting up, washing, eating and even socializing, which are imposed upon them. Many angry outbursts could be avoided by a patient-centred approach, which respects individual demands and negotiates individual needs.

Arguing with someone who is already angry is usually counter-productive. It is better to listen to their complaint, acknowledge their right to be angry (they usually have a good reason from their point of view), try to reach a negotiated settlement and, wherever possible, apologize. Early apologies usually elicit the response, 'Oh, it wasn't really your fault'. Try it next time a patient or superior expresses anger or discontent. However, much anger these days is encountered in situations where the individual concerned is under the influence of alcohol or drugs, and is therefore not behaving in a rational manner. In these situations, it is wise to back down and assume a submissive posture. Summon help or escape as soon as possible, but don't provoke an attack in the process.

Personal characteristics associated with stress

People are very different in how they perceive and experience events. What makes one person more resilient than another? This section introduces some of the relatively stable coping styles (personality factors). For more details, you may refer to Cooper and Payne (1991) and Miller (1992). It should be noted that, although these are described as relatively stable, it does not imply that they are not amenable to change.

Behaviour patterns

There has been a huge amount of research about the role of stress in the causation of heart disease, including large-scale epidemiological studies. Basically, it has been suggested that the characteristics of some people's personality may make them more vulnerable to developing coronary heart disease (CHD). The Type A behaviour pattern consists of three features (Friedman and Rosenman 1974):

1 Exaggerated sense of *time urgency*.
2 Excessive *competitiveness*, marked by a drive for achievement.
3 *Hostility* and *aggressiveness*.

People who display these characteristics have been found to be at greater risk of developing CHD, compared with people who show a Type B behaviour pattern. People with a Type B behaviour pattern do not demonstrate Type A features and are generally described as more easy-going and relaxed about life. These characteristics have been measured using a self-report questionnaire, which does not result in very good correlations with

CHD, and a structured interview (the Jenkins Activity Survey), which is a rather better measure, as it assesses responses which people are unaware of like fast speech and a tendency to interrupt, and other behaviours which people may not wish to acknowledge like aggressiveness. Most of the early research concentrated on men. It is possible that this is a culturally defined behaviour pattern, since punctuality, assertiveness (the desire to be in control) and competitiveness are all necessary and desirable attributes for employment success, especially in business in Western countries. The significance of a Type A behaviour pattern remains controversial, and current thinking suggests that other possible causes of heart disease and hypertension might involve the suppression of feelings of hostility, anger and aggression.

Exercise

Think of a situation in which you have felt very angry, but felt it necessary not to show this. Imagine how you felt and think about the effects on your heart rate, breathing rate and muscle tension. How did you calm down after this?

A Type C behaviour pattern, which may be associated with cancer proneness, has been described (Temoshok 1987). The Type C responses are passivity, compliance and suppression of anger. This could be thought to describe the perfect patient who never challenges medical authority! There is some evidence from research with breast cancer and lymphoma patients that excessive emotional control, especially in relation to the expression of anger, is as damaging to long-term survival prospects as excessive aggression is in CHD (Morris *et al.* 1992).

Hardiness

Kobasa (1979) introduced the concept of hardiness as a personality characteristic which has three components:

1 *Commitment* – an active involvement in life activities.
2 *Control* – a belief in the ability to influence life events.
3 *Challenge* – a belief that change is normal and growth-enhancing.

These factors are thought to be protective. Kobasa found that business executives who demonstrated these characteristics had low rates of illness. In a nursing study conducted in the United States by Nicholas (1993), elderly people who reported higher levels of hardiness perceived themselves to be fitter than others. In addition, it was found that people scoring high on hardiness were more likely to engage in good self-care behaviours. As more elderly people live alone in the community, it is important for their own welfare that they maintain or establish lifestyles that enhance their health, such as eating an adequate diet and preventing hypothermia. A greater awareness by nurses of the potential contribution of elderly people's personality styles, including hardiness, could be used to empower their clients.

Self-efficacy

Social learning theory (Bandura 1977) emphasizes various factors which are relevant to health behaviours, including the role of modelling in the acquisition of new health behaviours, the development of appropriate skills and self-efficacy, the belief that such changes are possible. Perceived self-efficacy is the conviction that one can successfully execute the behaviour required to produce a desired outcome. This moves from a simplistic view that information provision is sufficient to change behaviours. It is apparent that people often do not behave optimally, even though they know full well what to do. This is because self-referent thought mediates the relationship between knowledge and action (see the Theory of Planned Action in Chapter 2). Efficacy in dealing with one's environment is not a fixed act nor simply a matter of knowing what to do. Rather, it involves cognitive, social and behavioural skills which are integrated into courses of action. Perceived self-efficacy is concerned with judgements of how well one can execute courses of action. Self-efficacy judgements, whether accurate or faulty, influence choice of activities and environmental settings. People avoid activities that they believe exceed their coping capabilities, but they undertake and perform with confidence those that they judge themselves capable of managing. Judgements of self-efficacy also determine how much effort they will expend and how long they will persist in the face of obstacles or aversive experiences.

Personal control and locus of control

There has been a great deal of research using the concept of control (see Chapter 4), which does appear to be an important factor in understanding the relationship between stressful experience, behaviour and health. It appears that people who have an internal locus of control are more likely to engage in health screening and other health care behaviours, perhaps because they believe that these behaviours might make some difference. However, there may be some situations where it is unrealistic for people not to believe in the role of powerful others. For example, some individuals fail to report to the doctor until it is too late to receive help because they prefer to deal with the problem themselves. Patients with chronic kidney failure need regular medical interventions like haemodialysis and will die if they fail to place their trust in those who care for them. Research by Hack et al. (1994) found that women with breast cancer vary in their wishes to be involved in medical treatment decisions. Those women who wanted to play an active part desired detailed explanations about their disease and treatment options, but those patients who wished to be more passive and let their doctors decide on treatment were more likely to prefer less discussion about their illness. In terms of perceived control, they preferred that medical decisions were made by their doctors and these wishes need to be identified and respected. These wishes can only be found out about through individual negotiation.

If locus of control is based upon past experience, it may change with current and future experiences. Until recently, the health care system encouraged patients to believe in the power of doctors and to do as they were told (compliance). Raps *et al.* (1982) demonstrated that even short periods of hospitalization lead to identifiable cognitive, behavioural and emotional deficits. They suggested that the passive, compliant and inanimate behaviour which is often associated with the 'good patient' may actually be the result of learned helplessness. Nowadays, the emphasis is on 'empowerment' (increasing personal control) and patients are encouraged to engage in 'self-care'.

Exercise

Identify a client or patient you are currently caring for and carefully consider the intrapersonal factors discussed in this chapter. Identify the factors that may influence their health or recovery. What can you do, as a health professional, to enhance the outcomes for recovery and health?

The relationship between psychological concepts and interventions

A hypothetical model of the dynamic cycle of relationships between many of the concepts outlined in this chapter is illustrated in Fig. 6.4. In reality, people rarely find themselves in an extreme virtuous or vicious cycle, but fluctuate somewhere between the two, in a state of interdependence. The models of psychology outlined in Chapter 1 may be differentiated here by their priorities for intervention.

Stress in the work environment

Most of this chapter has been centred around the needs of patients or clients. However, it is necessary to recognize that stress is a normal daily occurrence and that caring for patients in the context of any organization, but particularly an NHS structure, is stressful. Bosses may be supportive or unsupportive (you may wish to look at the section on leadership in Chapter 9). As a result, you may feel valued or exploited. Some of the physical and mental symptoms of stress are identified below. You may wish to check to see if you can identify them in yourself from time to time:

- lack of appetite *or* eating too much
- feeling upset and crying

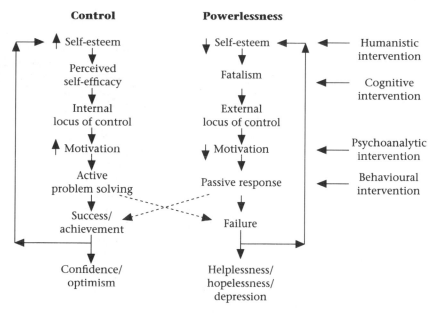

Figure 6.4 Hypothetical model of the dynamic relationships between control-related concepts and outcomes, with potential foci for intervention (Walker, J.M., previously unpublished).

- indigestion or nausea
- irritability and unreasonable behaviour
- feeling a failure
- difficulty in making decisions
- loss of sense of humour
- panic attacks or unreasonable fears
- tendency to take time off for minor illnesses
- tendency to use alcohol or nicotine to improve well-being

Stress is often associated with the high-flying executive (such as the Trust unit manager), but research demonstrates that physical and mental illness associated with stress is more common among blue-collar workers and those who have little control over their work. The structure of the organization often determines how much responsibility and support those at the coal face, or those involved in direct patient care, receive. When things go wrong, it is often these individuals who are blamed for their inability to cope, whereas in reality it is an organizational problem in which poor communication and lack of participation in decision making are important features. Where this is the case, it may be the 'sick' organization which requires assessment and change and not the 'sick' individual who needs counselling.

Health care has been through a period of rapid change in which individuals at all levels are experiencing uncertainty, unpredictability and uncontrollability to varying degrees. These problems are compounded when staff have their own personal, financial or health problems and lack support outside the work environment. The problem of **burnout** has long been recognized among the caring professions. This is where stress leads to low job satisfaction, poor performance and a lack of ability to empathize with patients. Tasks become ritualized and there is an increasing tendency to 'depersonalize' patients (see Chapter 9). Absence rates rise. Support groups for staff are an increasingly popular method of supporting carers, but these should be aimed at providing short-term emotional release and taking a constructive approach to improving the work environment. Leadership style, organizational structure and communication, and the management of change are important factors in generating or reducing stress within organizations. These are referred to again in Chapter 9.

Students are encouraged to recognize their own symptoms of stress, identify the sources of these and take appropriate action to deal with the problem appropriately at an early stage. Cooper *et al.* (1988) provide a useful guide to assist in this process.

A summary of the issues covered in this chapter is illustrated in Table 6.2.

Summary

- Response-based models of stress emphasize the common physiological consequences of stressful encounters.

- Stimulus-based models of stress emphasize the role of stressors in the environment.

- Transactional models of stress emphasize the role of cognitive processing in the appraisal and coping responses.

- Anxiety and depression are normal responses to uncertainty, unpredictability and uncontrollability.

- Psychological preparation is used to help people cope with medical procedures.

- Interpersonal factors like social support influence the way stress affects health.

- Intrapersonal factors like a Type A behaviour pattern, hardiness, self-efficacy and perceived control mediate the experience of stress and health outcomes.

- Stress affects everyone and is prevalent in organizations such as the NHS, which are undergoing a period of rapid change or suffer from poor communication networks.

Further reading

Bailey, R. and Clarke, M. (1989) *Stress and Coping in Nursing*. London: Chapman and Hall.

Table 6.2 Common factors related to stress formation and stress reduction (Walker, J.M., previously unpublished).

Environmental factors	Mediating factors	Common responses	Intervention principles
Catastrophic events Major life events Illness, disability and hospital treatment Daily hassles Organizational structure and management Sociopolitical factors (unemployment, poverty)	Individual coping styles: • perceived self-efficacy • locus of control • Type A/B/C pattern • hardiness Personal coping strategies: • active/passive • problem/emotion-focused Social support	Emotional and cognitive: • anxiety • depression • anger Behavioural: • adaptive/maladaptive Physical: • stress-related illness	Post-traumatic counselling and emotional support Inform, educate and provide resources for independence Teach coping strategies Better communication and involvement in decision making Increased sociopolitical involvement
Common factors are: Uncertainty Unpredictability Uncontrollability	Active problem solving promotes personal control Social support facilitates control	Loss of control is associated with cognitive, emotional and behavioural deficits (Seligman 1975) and disruption of homeostasis	*Aim:* reduce uncertainty, increase predictability, promote and facilitate control

Benner, P. and Wrubel, J. (1989) *The Primacy of Caring: Stress and Coping in Health and Illness*. Menlo Park, CA: Addison-Wesley. Chapters 2 and 3.

Cooper, C.L., Cooper, R.D. and Eaker, L.H. (1988) *Living with Stress*. Harmondsworth: Penguin.

Miller, J.F. (1992) *Coping with Chronic Illness: Overcoming Powerlessness*, 2nd edn. Philadelphia, PA: F.A. Davis. Chapter 2.

Oakley, A. (1992) *Social Support and Motherhood*. Oxford: Blackwell. Chapter 2.

Sarafino, E.P. (1994) *Health Psychology: Biopsychosocial Interactions*, 2nd edn. New York: John Wiley. Chapters 3–5.

Taylor, S.E. (1991) *Health Psychology*, 2nd edn. New York: McGraw-Hill. Chapter 8.

CHAPTER SEVEN

DEVELOPMENT AND LOSS IN SOCIAL RELATIONSHIPS

Introduction

How and why do people form relationships with each other? What happens when relationships end? Chapter 6 identified the importance of social relationships in influencing health and well-being. We tend to think that the formation of relationships occurs mostly in the early part of life and that losses occur mostly in the latter years; however, elderly people form new relationships (e.g. with their grandchildren), while losses (such as that of a grandparent or a pet) are common in childhood. Nurses and other carers need to understand the processes involved in forming and losing relationships because:

1 Relationships are often disrupted by ill-health and medical treatment.
2 Clients with health problems may be experiencing concurrent losses which add to the stressfulness of their situation.
3 The experience of loss may, itself, create health problems.

Therefore, in interactions with clients of all ages it is helpful to understand the nature of their social relationships. This will enable us to reach a better understanding of their attitudes and their behaviour and prevent misinterpretations and misunderstandings.

This chapter will provide an account of how early relationships are established, with reference to Bowlby's theory of attachment. This will be applied in the context of caring for infants and children in hospital. Subsequent developments in attachment theory will be used to understand the effects of early relationships on later behaviour. A necessary consequence of human development is psychological separation from the family for independent adult life. This process of separation will be examined. The final part of the chapter will focus on irrevocable losses such as bereavement. The concept of loss is explored against the background of the theoretical models that have been proposed to understand the process. The potential roles of health professionals in the process of loss and adjustment are explained.

Social relationships involve emotional commitment; in fact, that is how they are defined. If we felt nothing, it would not be a relationship. All of us experience attachments and losses throughout our lives. All attachments are not necessarily good, nor losses bad. They challenge us and can be thought of as contributing to our personal growth. As health professionals, we are often involved in, or are witnesses to, people's struggles to understand transitions in their social relationships.

Attachment

There have been a number of different theories about how and why the first attachment relationships between baby and mother are formed. One behaviourist view suggested that an infant's hunger is reduced by the mother feeding the child (a **drive-reduction** hypothesis). Another proposed that the baby learns to associate good things with the mother, like food, comfort and cuddles, which are reinforcing (an **operant conditioning** hypothesis). This is sometimes termed the 'cupboard love' theory. The problem with these hypotheses is that babies form relationships with many people, not just those who feed them, and that these relationships, once formed, are very long-lasting. Furthermore, Harlow's famous experiments with Rhesus monkeys illustrated how a baby monkey preferred to cling for comfort to a cloth-covered substitute mother, even when milk could only be obtained from a wire substitute mother. There appears to be something more to the formation of social relationships than the availability of primary reinforcers. In fact, the theories which have made the greatest contribution to our current understanding of attachment in young children have emerged from the psychoanalytic tradition. This is probably because psychoanalytic psychologists have a preference for investigating the impact of close family relationships on psychological development.

Bowlby's theory of attachment

The currently accepted theory of early relationships was originally proposed by John Bowlby in the post-war period (see Bowlby 1969). Bowlby was influenced by psychoanalytic theory, by ethology (the study of animals in their natural habitat) and by his experience as a psychiatrist, working with difficult behaviour in adolescents. From psychoanalytic theory (see Chapter 1), he adopted notions of predetermined biological patterns of instinctive behaviour in the newborn infant, such as sucking and crying (to the demands of the id). From ethology, he derived the concept of **imprinting**, in which certain types of newborn animals demonstrate immediate and irreversible attachments. This concept was generalized to human beings as **bonding**, which will be described in more detail later. In his clinical work, Bowlby had noticed that adolescents with behavioural problems often had a history of poor care or disruption in their family during childhood.

Bowlby proposed that both infants and mothers have evolved a biological need to stay in constant contact with one another. This was likely to ensure the survival of infants, because they would be fed, protected from harm and loved. His theory had the following main hypotheses:

1 There is a **sensitive period** between birth and 5 years of age which is the optimal time for bonding.
2 **Attachment behaviours** are designed to bring the mother to the infant. These include crying or smiling or, when the infant is older, the child following or staying close to the mother.
3 The mother or other main care-giver is the **primary attachment figure**.
4 Infants establish an attachment with one person.
5 Once this attachment has occurred, the child will remain attached to that individual.

This is a summary of the theory of attachment which is based on an interactional model. Attachment is not dependent solely on the infant's or mother's responses; rather, both participants influence each other. Attachment is dependent upon a close and enduring relationship in early life. Therefore, a depressed mother who is unable to respond adequately to the infant's demands for attention, may influence the baby's subsequent behaviour by failing to respond to signals like crying. Likewise, a very small pre-term infant may be unable to produce the responses like crying or smiling which elicit adult attention. Bowlby has suggested that primary attachment is important in infancy because it provides the template for subsequent relationships. We need to experience positive feelings of love for one person to know how to love others. We learn about reciprocity, the give-and-take in social relationships. Moreover, without this loving early relationship, emotional development may become distorted. Bowlby emphasized that separation from the primary care-giver before the age of 5 years might damage the mental health of the child. Harlow demonstrated that Rhesus monkeys deprived of all contact with their mothers and other Rhesus monkeys during their development showed no affection for their own babies and tended to abuse them physically. It has been suggested that psychopaths, people who show no understanding of the feelings of others or guilt if they hurt others, may lack experience of early attachments. Another reason why attachment formation is vital, is that it enables children to feel secure enough to start to explore their environment, which is essential for cognitive development. The details of how attachment occurs are considered below, together with the extent to which Bowlby's original ideals have been supported by more recent research.

The development of attachment (adapted from Berk 1991)

1 *The pre-attachment phase* (birth to 6 weeks). Immediately after birth, the infant has reflex responses, such as sucking, rooting (turning the head towards the breast to suckle) and grasping. Although these reflexes disappear over the first few weeks, they have obvious survival functions. Newborn infants seem to be very much oriented towards other humans. Although they have relatively poor eyesight compared with adults, they prefer to look at human faces rather than other objects (Goren *et al.* 1975). They seem to be comforted more by human voices than music. They are able to recognize their own mother's voice and her smell. It seems that healthy infants arrive in the world equipped with responses which elicit the attention of adults. It is very difficult to ignore a crying baby and most people find their responses rewarding. So although irreversible attachment may not yet have taken place, the infant's behaviours and adults' responses seem to prepare for continuing social relationships.

2 *The 'attachment-in-the-making' phase* (6 weeks to 6–8 months). Babies start to smile at around 6 weeks and this proves very rewarding for adult care-givers. At about 6–8 months, the infant starts to show a definite preference for a particular person, usually the mother. Berk (1991) suggests that babies become upset by separation, although this includes other attachment figures and does not relate only to separation from the mother.

3 *The phase of established attachment* (6–8 months to 18–24 months). By this phase, babies demonstrate instant recognition of their mother. They appear able to hold a mental representation (like a picture in their head) of her when she is no longer present. This is termed 'object permanence', which is part of the theory of cognitive development described by Piaget, who emphasized how important it was for children to acquire the ability to know that things continue to exist, even when they are not present in the environment. Typically, infants of this age will show separation anxiety when their mother leaves. This involves protests like crying and searching for their mother. As children become more mobile by crawling and walking, these behaviours enable them to maintain contact with their mother and can make it difficult for her to leave them for even short periods.

4 *Formation of reciprocal relationship* (18–24 months and older). By this phase, children begin to use language to express their needs and negotiate

with their mother and other carers. For example, if they are lost or frightened, they call for their mother. Separation anxiety declines as the child learns more about the mother's behaviour and is able to predict, under familiar circumstances, when she will return.

Separation

Robertson made a series of harrowing films which revealed the extent and characteristics of distress shown by separated young children. The stages were:

- *Protest* – marked by anger and loud crying.
- *Despair* – marked by withdrawal and less vigorous crying.
- *Detachment* – marked by an outward display of cheerful behaviour but the child remained emotionally distant.

These children showed inappropriate social behaviour by approaching strange adults but did not establish emotional contact with them. Even when reunited with their parents, these children displayed ambivalent and disturbed behaviours like pushing their mother away or refusing to be held or cuddled.

Bowlby's theory has been very influential in changing the way that children are cared for in hospitals, obstetric units and by social services in Britain and other Western countries. In the past, it was common for young children to be separated, deliberately, from their parents on admission to hospital or when they were placed in residential care.

Evidence for the three main elements of Bowlby's theory – bonding, attachment behaviours and primary attachment figure – are considered below.

'Bonding'

Observational research carried out by ethologists, who study animals in their natural habitat, discovered that certain species experience a process called 'imprinting'. Konrad Lorenz discovered, by accident, that in the first 24 hours after hatching, greylag geese chicks follow, and form an attachment to, the first moving object they see (in the wild this is invariably the parent geese). In species where it is necessary for the infant to follow the parent to find or obtain food, and where the offspring are mobile immediately after birth, this type of 'imprinting' behaviour is necessary for survival. In mammals such as goats and sheep, it was observed that the mother would reject her infant if she was denied the immediate opportunity to lick it clean. These needs in birds and animals for immediate contact were subsequently generalized to human beings as the need for 'bonding'. Kennel et al. (1979) emphasized the need for the mother to have close physical 'skin-to-skin' contact immediately after birth with her newborn in order to promote bonding and attachment between mother and infant. It was thought that type of contact was necessary if successful mothering was to occur. A correlation was observed between babies with a low birthweight, requiring care in a special care baby unit, and subsequent abuse.

The concept of bonding has become very influential. Women are now encouraged to have skin-to-skin contact with their newborn babies immediately after delivery. However, there is very little research evidence that 'bonding' is a biological requirement in humans. First, human infants are not mobile and therefore cannot wander off. Second, it implies that mothers who do not immediately feel love for their newborns are somehow abnormal, whereas attachment between mothers and infants often occurs over the first few weeks of life. Third, if bonding was a biological imperative that had to occur immediately after birth, this would imply that babies ·could only form attachments to their biological mother. However, there is plenty of evidence that attachments can be made with adoptive parents some considerable time later. Therefore, it is possible to reassure mothers whose very sick babies need immediate resuscitation and medical care after birth, that they will still be able to form good relationships with their child. Studies of children who have suffered social deprivation and been institutionalized indicate that they are able to form stable attachments even in middle childhood (Hodges and Tizard 1989). The notion of a sensitive period for 'bonding' may be true, but it is considerably longer than was proposed by Kennel *et al*. In fact, the concept of immediate bonding may induce guilt in mothers who do not feel an immediate surge of maternal feeling and could impose undue pressure on mothers whose relationship with their babies is naturally slow to develop.

Attachment behaviour

It certainly seems that babies have evolved to provide cues that elicit adult attention and care-giving. Babies have facial characteristics, such as large wide set eyes, wide cheeks and short faces, which adults find appealing (Alley 1981). These cues have been exploited by cartoon and film makers, as in *Bambi* and *ET*. Attachment behaviours are based on reciprocal interactions. The mother and the infant influence each other's responses. Detailed observations of the interaction between a mother and her baby reveal a synchronization between the behaviour of the baby, such head-turning, looking, smiling or arm movements, and the verbal responses of the mother. There appears to be a turn-taking, which is thought to teach infants the basic patterns of behaviour which will later become the turn-taking of conversation. This is a very subtle social skill, but one which is vital to the formation and maintenance of successful social relationships later on. Interactions develop in complexity over the first 6 months and may be seen in games like 'pat-a-cake' and 'peek-a-boo'. Care-givers need to monitor their interactions carefully so they do not over-stimulate the infant. It has been noted that many adults automatically use a special type of slowed and simplified speech, called 'motherese', when interacting with babies. It seems reasonable to assume that a mother or primary care-giver, who is totally emotionally committed to the welfare and well-being of the child, will be better able to develop a mutually rewarding reciprocal relationship with the child than someone who does not feel this sense of commitment. Attachment behaviours on both sides of the interaction are equally important. Excessive crying or a failure to respond on the part of the child may be as disruptive in the development of this relationship as a lack of commitment and attention on the part of the care-giver.

Primary attachment figure

Bowlby emphasized the importance of a primary attachment figure. He thought it would usually be the biological mother, although he did acknowledge that it could be a substitute care-giver. Subsequent research has shown that children may form a particularly strong attachment to one person, although this is not always with the mother, and children often form multiple attachments. Fathers, siblings and 'significant' others can also be attachment figures, depending upon the social circumstances of the child (Schaffer and Emerson 1964). Children also form attachments to pets and inanimate objects like teddy bears and blankets. Approximately 50 per cent of 2- and 3-year-olds are strongly attached to a soft toy or blanket (Passman and Halonen 1979). Children use such an object as a form of reassurance in strange or frightening situations, like a hospital. When caring for young children, it is helpful to suggest that they bring a teddy or other favourite soft toy with them to the ward or clinic. Overall, it seems to be protective for children to have a hierarchy of attachment figures, whether they have a preferred attachment or not, because these ensure that they can be comforted by other people or things that they know and trust.

Attitudes to parenting

Attitudes to parenting vary according to the historical and cultural context of the time. For instance, throughout most of this century in Britain it has been socially and morally acceptable to inflict physical punishment on children. This was embodied in sayings such as 'spare the rod, and spoil the child'. However, over the past decade, physical punishment is no longer perceived to be acceptable in schools and is condemned by many as a form of punishment for use in the home. This influence has come from sources as diverse as human rights organizations, humanist psychologists and behaviourists such as B.F. Skinner. There are other major differences in child care practices across the world. For example, there tends to be more physical contact in Third World countries than in the West because mothers tend to carry their baby's everywhere they go. Does breast-feeding confer any long-term psychological advantage (as opposed to physiological advantage) over bottle-feeding? Are there any differences in children who grow up to experience communal types of care, such as those afforded by the extended family, a kibbutz or nursery, compared with those who grow up in a close intimate environment of a nuclear or single-parent family? The existence of substantial differences in patterns of child-rearing may serve to illustrate how resilient and adaptable the human infant is. However, it is interesting to speculate how these variations in parenting might have influenced child and adult development.

Exercise

Look at a selection of baby-care advice books for mothers. How do they describe the 'best' type of care? For example, do they recommend demand or time-schedule feeding? Breast- or bottle-feeding? What recommendations are made about controlling or punishing 'naughty' behaviour? Is some of the advice contradictory? What does it say about current values and morals? If you can, try to find baby books from earlier on this century, or from other countries, and compare the advice given. Is it possible to establish which advice is right and which is wrong?

Measurement of attachment

The most common experimental method of measuring attachment is the 'Strange Situation' (Ainsworth *et al.* 1978). This is an experimental procedure (see Table 7.1) which aims to identify the type of attachment shown by the child. The procedure elicits separation anxiety responses and careful observations are made of how the child and mother interact before and after separation episodes. The original observations took place with 14-month-old children of middle-class American mothers. The following types of attachment were identified:

1 *Secure attachment* (approximately 66 per cent). These children were happy to explore the environment when their mother was present. They might

Table 7.1 Measuring the security of attachment (adapted from Ainsworth *et al.* 1978).

Persons present	Duration	Events
1. Mum + baby	30 seconds	Experimenter in room
2. Mum + baby	3 minutes	Mother plays with baby
3. Mum + baby + stranger	3 minutes	Stranger enters room
4. Stranger + baby	3 minutes	Mum leaves
5. Mum + baby	3 minutes	Mum returns
6. Baby alone	3 minutes	Mum leaves
7. Stranger + baby	3 minutes	Stranger enters
8. Mum + baby	3 minutes	Mum returns

cry on separation, but on her return they sought immediate contact with her and crying was immediately reduced.

2 *Avoidant attachment* (approximately 20 per cent). These children showed no distress at separation with their mother. When she returned, they did not rush to greet her and avoided contact, although they did not resist physical contact.

3 *Resistant attachment* (approximately 10–12 per cent). These children were thought to show ambivalent responses. They stayed close to their mother before separation, and were very distressed by her leaving the room. But when she returned they appeared to be angry with her, hitting and pushing at her, and continued to cry even when offered physical comfort.

4 *Disorganized/disoriented attachment* (approximately 5 per cent). The last category was identified by Main and Soloman (1986). These children appear to be very confused and show contradictory responses, like approaching their mother, but with no signs of pleasure.

The 'Strange Situation' is widely used to measure the types of attachment shown by children. However, it is necessary to be cautious about presuming that only secure attachments are 'normal'. There is in fact considerable variability in what can be considered normal relationships and responses. For example, observations in Germany and Japan indicate that they are quite different from the American pattern. It seems likely that parents make different demands on their children depending upon individual differences and what is considered to be 'normal' in each culture.

Attachment theory has highlighted the detrimental effects of maternal deprivation and institutionalized care for young children. The most damaging aspects are the use of multiple care-givers who are unable to engage in long-term emotionally rewarding relationships with the individual child. This denies such children the opportunity to develop or experience secure attachments. There is evidence that children with insecure attachment fail to do well in school and have difficulties in forming relationships with other children. There is much less evidence about the long-term consequences for adult mental health, largely because it is difficult to establish the nature of early relationships in retrospect, while longitudinal studies are rare because they are expensive and difficult to undertake. Although adults who have mental health problems may have had disrupted early relationships, they are also likely to have experienced other adverse conditions such as poverty, poor housing and inadequate education (Rutter 1981). It is also possible that differences in attachment could be accounted for by the child's temperament. Thus difficult and fussy children may be less responsive to parenting behaviours than easy-going, contented and happy children, and in turn are less rewarding or more challenging to care for. It is difficult to conclude on the basis of the present evidence that insecure attachments cause mental illness in adulthood. Failure to form attachments is an important feature of autism. Parents frequently report that they fail to make eye contact or respond to close physical contact or affection. Autism may be caused by a genetic defect and autistic children often have additional learning difficulties.

The influence of attachment theory on the care of sick children has been profound. Children are no longer routinely separated from their parents on admission to hospital. Ideally, children are cared for by specially trained staff (Price 1994), within areas of the hospital specially adapted to meet their physical, emotional and intellectual needs. There has been a consistent attempt to provide care for children which does not involve separation, such as day-case surgery and the appointment of specially trained community paediatric nurses to provide care at home. However, there remain a number of children, particularly those with chronic diseases, who experience repeated admissions to hospital or who need regular medical supervision (Eiser 1993). In these cases, the mother is encouraged to remain with the child to provide care and emotional support. However, it is worth noting that this can result in feelings of deprivation on the part of a well sibling who remains at home in the care of the father, relatives or friends. This can result in difficult choices for families, particularly when their home is not close to the unit in which the sick child is being treated.

Life transitions

During normal development over the lifespan, people need to separate from some social relationships and develop new ones. Children leave their parents to go to school and develop new relationships with teachers and peers. An important later period of transition takes place in adolescence and early adulthood, when people establish their own identity and form new types of relationships with peers. It is at this stage that the first intimate sexual relationships (heterosexual or homosexual) occur. Erikson (1963) developed an eight-stage model of psychosocial development (see Table 7.2). His ideas were developed from psychoanalytic theory. Erikson emphasized that at each stage of development there are special issues that must be confronted (called crises) before development can proceed successfully. For example, in the first year of life, the baby needs to develop a trusting relationship with another person, usually the mother; and if the relationship is established, that is considered to be a successful outcome. This is rather similar to the attachment process that Bowlby proposed.

SPECIAL TOPIC

Teenage motherhood

The Health of the Nation (DoH 1992a) document highlighted the increasing trend for young women under 20 years of age to become mothers. It has become a public health target to reduce the rates of pregnancy in this age group. There are known to be increased obstetric risks to the mother and a higher incidence of low birthweight in babies born to very young women. Teenage motherhood is also associated with economic and social problems. When compared with older mothers, teenagers show poorer parenting skills, such as being more restrictive and less sensitive to their babies' needs. If we take a developmental perspective, adolescence and parenthood are both associated with major transitions. In Britain, developmental tasks in

Table 7.2 Erikson's eight stages of psychosocial development (adapted from Erikson 1963).

Stages	Psychosocial crises	Significant social relationships	Favourable outcome
1. First year of life	Trust vs mistrust	Mother or mother substitute	Trust and optimism
2. Second year	Autonomy vs doubt	Parents	Sense of self-control and adequacy
3. Third to fifth years	Initiative vs guilt	Basic family	Purpose and direction
4. Sixth year to puberty	Industry vs inferiority	Neighbourhood, school	Competence in intellectual, social and physical skills
5. Adolescence	Identity vs confusion	Peer groups and outgroups; models of leadership	An integrated image of oneself as a unique person
6. Early adulthood	Intimacy vs isolation	Partners in friendship; sex, competition, cooperation	Ability to form close and lasting relationships; to make career commitments
7. Middle adulthood	Generativity vs self-absorption	Divided labour and shared household	Concern for family, society and future generations
8. The ageing years	Integrity vs despair	'Mankind', 'My kind'	A sense of fulfilment and satisfaction with one's life

adolescence include establishing an identity, obtaining an education and/or employment, and usually moving away from the family home. According to Erikson, developmental tasks in early adulthood include forming stable intimate relationships, rearing the next generation and establishing a career. When all these tasks face young mothers, how do they cope with the challenge? There may be dilemmas, such as whether they should complete their education and continue to live with their original family, or seek to establish their independence by moving into their own home.

In an American nursing research study by Spieker and Bensley (1994), 197 adolescent mother–infant pairs were assessed to identify to what extent the social support provided by the adolescents' mothers, and their living arrangements, influenced the type of attachment shown by the infants. As suggested in the last chapter, social support may help to modify the effects of stress. The results of this study showed that infants were more likely to be securely attached if their mothers lived with their partners and had a high level of social support from their own mothers. If the teenage parent's mother did not provide social support, then the infants seemed to do better when their mother lived independently, rather than with her partner. This is a rather complex study, but it indicates that there are disadvantages for the new baby if the teenage mother continues to live at home, although there are advantages for the new mother if she receives experienced help with child care. It is possible that in this situation it is difficult for a young mother to display parenting behaviours towards her child in the presence of her own mother. In these circumstances, the baby may become confused as to whether it is the mother or grandmother who is the primary attachment figure. Of course, it probably requires an exceptional degree of emotional maturity for a teenager to establish a successful home with a partner, and maintain the goodwill of their mother, while caring for the demands of a baby. As this is a correlational study, it is impossible to distinguish between cause and effect.

Teenage motherhood presents challenges for health and social services. A developmental perspective shows how the needs of three generations may conflict: the maternal grandmother, the teenage mother and her partner, and the child. Less pessimistically, many young people adapt well to the demands of parenthood and it cannot be assumed that all teenage pregnancies are unplanned or unwanted.

Middle life represents a difficult transition for many adults. It is a time when children have grown up and are wanting to gain independence or leave home. Women must relinquish their role as mother and carer and find other means of fulfilment. Parents who have had little time for each other suddenly find themselves spending more time in each other's company. Men and women have to confront the fact that they may never fulfil their life-long ambitions and many face early retirement with little to look forward to. Retirement is an important transition for both partners. If the woman has remained at home, she may find her partner's continual presence an unwelcome intrusion. The person who has retired, whether man or woman, may find themselves bored and suffer from loss of esteem and depression if they have no other activities to keep themselves involved or stimulated.

In later life, Erikson proposed that people attain a sense of fulfilment or despair. The Erikson model has been particularly useful in trying to understand the experiences and needs of elderly people, a group who had been much neglected within psychology. For example, it has stimulated interest in reminiscence and life-review therapy with elderly people who require institutional care. Haight (1988) developed a protocol for 6 one-hour life-review sessions which could be used by professional and lay carers to help elderly people attain a sense of psychological well-being. They were encouraged during these sessions to recount important events from their childhood and adulthood and to review these in a positive light. These sessions helped them to validate their past experiences, share pride in past achievements, and assert their individuality.

Exercise

Talk to an elderly person about the way they feel about their life. How might you describe their psychosocial development in terms of Erikson's theory? Do you think that they have made a successful transition into old age or are there any factors which you think might be hindering successful adaptation? Do you feel that Erikson's model is useful in understanding these issues? Can you identify other theories (for example, see Chapter 6) which might help to account for any current problems that this person has?

Erikson's model has been criticized for being rather vague, in that it is difficult to know how to assess the adequacy of psychosocial outcomes. For instance, how can we know whether or not 'trust' has been established in babies? Nevertheless, Erikson's model is useful to health professionals because it reminds us of the integration of psychological and social elements in an individual's life. It also reminds us that development is a life-long process.

Loss, grief and mourning

Throughout life, we experience losses. We need to come to terms with these losses and integrate them with our continuing life, or our mental health may suffer. Experiencing loss is an inevitable part of life. When we make choices about careers, relationships, or places and ways to live, one choice is often mutually incompatible with another. Therefore, choosing one may mean the loss of the other. Transitions like marriage or promotion at work bring both gains and losses. Some losses may not be of actual things or events, but of potential events, roles or relationships, and it is therefore possible to lose something that you have never had. This is a type of loss which is experienced by many infertile couples, for whom the role of parent cannot be realized. Other losses, like unemployment, home-lessness or loss of a body part or function, are more obvious. Finally, the majority of us will experience the deaths of people we love, and all of us face the finality of our own death. It has been suggested that one of the reasons why some health professionals choose to work with people who are suffering and ill is because they fear their own death, and this may be why they appear to experience a particularly high degree of death anxiety. You may speculate about the sources of the assumptions underlying this assertion.

The next section describes and considers theories which account for people's experience of loss. The implications of these theories for health care practice will be considered. It is first necessary to define the basic terms. **Bereavement** is a process surrounding the loss of a loved object. This is usually a person, but may be a pet, a job, a way of life, a belief system, or in fact anything which has personal meaning for us. **Grief** is the reaction associated with such a loss.

Grief has many components and is best thought of as a holistic response to loss. Grief is a normal process; it is not a state nor probably even a series of stages. Grief is painful. It affects almost all aspects of a person. The emotional symptoms of grief include depression, anxiety, guilt, anger, loneliness and loss of enjoyment of life. There are behavioural changes which include restlessness, tiredness and crying. Psychological changes associated with grief may include low self-esteem, helplessness, hope-lessness, or a sense of unreality or denial. A person may be preoccupied with the deceased person and experience yearning, ambivalence, idealiza-tion or imitation. It may be very difficult to think clearly or concentrate. Grief also affects physical function with a possible loss of appetite, insomnia and lethargy. People describe grief as physically painful, and they may need reassurance that they are not ill. In addition, people may cope with their grief by increasing their use of mood-altering substances like alcohol, tobacco or drugs. These impede successful adaptation and contribute an added risk to health. It is known that there is an increased risk of death for widowers in the first few years after the death of their spouse. People appear to be more susceptible to infections, certain diseases, accidents and suicide after a bereavement. It is thought that immunological depression contributes to this increase in morbidity and mortality. Health profession-als need to be aware that bereaved people are potentially vulnerable. It may be helpful to encourage people to share their feelings and to let them know that these are a normal part of grieving. We cannot take their pain away but we can offer them support and understanding.

Mourning is the behavioural and emotional expression of grief. Mourn-ing is influenced strongly by cultural norms. For example, the rituals that occur after a death, such as laying out the body, the type of funeral and type of clothing worn by mourners, are all very much dependent upon the culture in which one lives. In America, it is common practice to have open coffins, whereas this is very uncommon in Britain. In Ireland, where communities are small and intimate, the funeral is often followed by a communal celebration, or wake, while in Britain a small family gathering is more common, in which the deceased individual is remembered in the context of family traditions and activities. It is probably helpful to have well-accepted rituals because they direct people how to behave and how to respond to each other during a time when it is difficult to make informed decisions. Rituals, such as state funerals, both contain and allow public expression of feelings. They also mark the status change of individuals, such as a wife becoming a widow. They provide an opportunity to demonstrate emotional support, and enable grieving people to derive comfort from others. Nurses engage in ritualized care after the death of a patient; the body is laid out in a manner that has changed little over the last century (Wolf 1986). Many nurses describe this final act of care as very important in showing respect for the person they have cared for, and in providing themselves with a sense of completion (Lawler 1991).

Exercise

Describe the mourning practices in the community or culture in which you have grown up. Think about the following questions. How do people dress? Are they allowed/expected to cry in public? Are there gender differences in permitted expressions of emotion? How do religious beliefs influence these practices? How long do people mourn for? Try to compare your description with a colleague from another country, ethnic or religious group.

Theories of loss

Most theories of **loss**, like attachment, have been derived from a psychoanalytic perspective, simply because the key theorists in this area have emerged from that tradition. Central to these theories is the concept of 'ego defence', which means that some things which happen to people may be so threatening that the conscious mind, the ego, cannot cope with them. Freud introduced the notion of defence mechanisms, which are unconscious ways of coping, like denial. It is suggested that we all use these mechanisms but in an unconscious way. Moreover, they may be helpful in allowing us to continue functioning in very stressful situations, and later we can 'work through' (consciously process) threatening feelings. Freud suggested that to recover from loss we need to confront our fears and feelings in a conscious manner which he called 'grief work'. Failure to do this, he thought, might lead to prolonged or pathological types of grief.

Attachment theory conceptualizes grief as a form of separation anxiety (Bowlby 1980). Thus the same pattern of protest, despair and detachment described by Robertson may be seen in loss. These responses appear to be triggered by the loss of an attachment figure. The closer and stronger the attachment, the more intense and enduring the response. This theory predicts that we would be considerably more distressed by the loss of one's spouse than a distant cousin. Interestingly, those who have experienced a happy and fulfilled marriage sometimes find it easier to adjust to widowhood than those who experienced an unhappy or unfulfilled relationship. Can you find an explanation for this?

Kubler-Ross (1969) described a *stage model of loss* based on her clinical experiences with dying patients. She described how patients who were given a life-threatening diagnosis, like cancer, appeared to pass through five stages before reaching psychological adjustment:

1 **Denial**. According to Kubler-Ross (1969: 34), an initial reaction to being given a terminal prognosis is typically, 'No, not me, it cannot be true'. People reject the reality of the situation and search for more comforting explanations of their symptoms.
2 **Anger**. After a while, there is a realization that the diagnosis is true. Then reactions like 'anger, rage, envy and resentment' (p. 44) are experienced. People may become very critical of nursing and medical care during this stage.
3 **Bargaining**. People try to negotiate with their carers, God or others for more time, relief from pain or suffering. There is little logic to these attempts, just a desperate desire to alter the course of events. At this stage, patients may seek a range of treatments at different centres.
4 **Depression**. As the course of the disease progresses, the impact of loss is expressed as depression. There may be multiple losses throughout the disease; for instance, in laryngeal cancer, initial surgery may remove the voice or alter it, which may mean loss of employment and changes in social contact. Increasing weakness may mean changes to a person's ability to be an active parent or spouse. Therefore, the individual may be grieving for the actual losses that have already occurred and those that they anticipate in the future. A common aspect of depression is withdrawal from contact with family and friends.
5 **Acceptance**. If there is sufficient time in the course of dying, the person may achieve a quiet calm understanding of their fate. For some, this is within the context of a belief system like religion, which provides an explanation of their life and hope for a future.

The model has become very popular with nurses and other caring professionals. However, although 'Kubler-Ross' stages provide a framework to understand adjustment to loss, there is little evidence that people necessarily experience all these stages, and certainly not in the order presented. Reactions to loss are very variable. Individuals often experience considerable ambivalence and mood swings. It is often unhelpful to categorize dying people in terms of stages. An alternative is to regard the process of dying as yet another life transition which presents challenges to us. How we cope with the challenges will depend on many factors, including previous personality, our social relationships and the support we have, the nature of our disease and symptoms, and the quality of care we receive.

Perhaps the most powerful feelings of loss most of us will experience are associated with the death of a loved one. Parkes (1986) developed a model of loss occurring after a bereavement. He has suggested that all significant losses result in a major and rapid change to people's taken-for-granted world, which is threatening and frightening. The following processes have been proposed:

1 Numbness and disbelief.
2 An initial alarm reaction, which is experienced as anxiety, restlessness and fear.
3 Searching (which is similar to Bowlby's ideas of yearning and protest).
4 Pining, which Parkes (1986: 61) describes as 'A persistent and obtrusive wish for the person who is gone, a preoccupation with thoughts that can only give pain'. He suggests that pining is the emotional expression of searching.
5 Mitigating and avoiding the pain of grief by continuing to interact with the deceased, such as feeling their presence and talking to them.
6 Anger and guilt.
7 Depression and withdrawal.
8 Feeling of loss of the self.
9 Identification with the lost person.
10 Resolution of grief.

As with the Kubler-Ross model, it is simplistic to think that everyone experiences all these responses and in this order. Grief is commonly experienced as acute painful pangs or episodes rather than as a continual state. There may be times such as birthdays, anniversaries of the death, or other special occasions like Christmas, when the grief is particularly acute. Grief can also be triggered by small events or reminders of the person. At one time it was thought that people recovered from bereavement in a matter of a few weeks or months. It is now known to be a much longer process, commonly lasting years, rather than months, although the intensity of distress diminishes over time. It is probably wrong to think of people 'recovering' from bereavement, since this suggests that they are ill and that once 'recovered' they will get back to normal life as it was before. First, grief is not an illness but a normal process. Second, losses change us and our world. We are never quite the same again, although this does not mean that we cannot form new relationships or enjoy life. So there is hope for the future and it can be comforting to share this with bereaved people without denying the impact of their loss. Very occasionally, people experience complicated or very prolonged grief reactions which may need specialist interventions, but the majority of people are very resilient and cope with loss using their own resources.

A recent alternative to the 'stage' models of loss has been proposed by Stroebe (1994). She suggested an 'oscillation' model in which the bereavement person is envisaged to swing between *loss orientation* and *future orientation*. These swings can occur at any time. During loss orienta- tion, the person will be displaying grieving behaviours such as crying and thinking about the lost person. It may be very difficult for them to focus on everyday activities like making a meal or going back to work. During future orientation, the person will be focused on everyday tasks such as caring for children and dealing with the family finances. It is anticipated that in the period immediately after a bereavement, more time will be spent in loss orientation than in future orientation, and the reverse would be true as time passes. However, events or memories might cause people to swing between these two orientations even many years later. Stroebe argues that abnormal bereavement outcomes might result from becoming 'stuck' in either of these orientations.

Loss of a pet

Many people, especially elderly people, have close relationships and attachments with their pets. Archer and Winchester (1994) surveyed 88 people in England to discover how they felt about the death of their pet dog or cat. They wanted to discover how distressing the loss of a pet was compared with a human bereavement. They found a similar pattern of grief to human losses, although with rather less emotional distress in most instances. Over half the respondents reported numbness and/or disbelief after the death of their pet, and found that they were preoccupied by thoughts of the animal.

Critical evaluation of the assumptions about coping with loss

Wortman and Silver (1989) have argued that there is little evidence for some of the assumptions made about **coping** with loss:

1 *Distress or depression is inevitable.* It is commonly assumed that everyone who experiences a loss will be distressed. However, in studies of be- reaved people, not everyone becomes depressed.
2 *Distress is necessary.* According to psychoanalytic theories of loss, such as those described above, people need to confront the reality of their loss before things can start to get better. In fact, if people do not show distress, it is thought to be indicative of pathology. Kubler-Ross suggests that depression occurs before acceptance. However, research with widows conducted by Vachon *et al.* (1982) indicated that those who were most depressed in the early stages were also the people most likely to be still depressed after 2 years.
3 *The importance of 'working through' feelings of loss.* It is assumed that resolution of grief requires cognitive-emotional processing and this is the aim of interventions like psychotherapy or bereavement counselling. Yet studies have shown that people who exhibit high levels of yearning or pining tend to have a poorer outcome in the long term, regardless of intervention.
4 *The expectation of recovery.* All models of loss assume that the final out- come of grieving will be a return to a normal psychological state, although the time-span is not generally specified. Wortman and Silver (1989) suggest that for a minority of individuals, grieving may continue over many years without it being abnormal. There are few research studies that have followed up people over many years, so it is difficult to know how long a 'normal' period of grieving lasts.
5 *Reaching a state of resolution.* It is commonly assumed that people will eventually reach a time when they are able to think and talk calmly about the loss without feeling undue distress. The person will have

established an understanding and reason (not necessarily a medical one) for the death. One of the ways health professionals can help bereaved people is to help them to find a meaning and purpose to explain why the person died. It is often more difficult to come to terms with a death which is unexplained, such as a miscarriage, stillbirth or cot death, or in which there is no body such as a drowning at sea. It seems that sudden deaths (e.g. in road traffic accidents) and untimely deaths (such as in children or young people) are very difficult for the bereaved to come to terms with.

Many families are now spread geographically, so that they see each other only seldom. In these circumstances, the grieving process may not follow the 'normal' pattern. A friend who saw her family only about four times a year, reported that the loss of her mother did not sink in until about 4 months after the funeral, at which time a visit was overdue. From that point, the grief became stronger as there was no-one around who knew her mother and with whom she could share reminiscences about her. Acceptance took many years and there are still episodes of strong emotional distress and guilt that she was not present to share her mother's dying.

Exercise

(If you have recently experienced a bereavement you may prefer not to do this exercise.)
Think about a loss you have experienced in the past (e.g. the loss of a pet, a grandparent, a patient, etc.). Write down your reactions. Try to remember how you became aware of the death. What did you do? How did you feel? What were your reactions after 3 months, 6 months, 1 year, 2 years? How clearly can you remember the way you felt at each time? How much did this loss interfere with your life? You may like to compare these experiences with a friend or colleague, which will give you an insight into how different individual grief reactions are.

Anticipatory grief

Some time after the death of her father, a young woman returned to the hospital ward on which he died to thank the nursing staff. She explained that, despite the distress and pain she experienced when informed of her father's terminal condition and his subsequent death, she was grateful for the time period between these two events. Amongst other things, it gave her time to resolve conflicts, express her love and say goodbye.

(Evans 1994: 160)

This story suggests that we are able to help people prepare for the bereavement period and start to mourn their loss before the death has actually occurred. Much of the care offered to relatives of dying patients is based on the assumption that 'grief work' can begin prior to the death. It is thought to be helpful for relatives to face up to this imminent loss, and the grief experienced then will help to prevent subsequent abnormal bereavement. However, the research evidence about anticipatory grief is rather confused. Evans (1994) has suggested that instead of focusing on the death, we should be aware of the multiple losses that occur for patients and their carers during a terminal illness.

Alzheimer's disease illustrates a protracted series of losses that must be faced by a spouse. For example, a wife loses the person she once married; the friend, social companion, lover; the income-provider; the car driver; the person to argue with; and so on. These losses may occur gradually over the years, each loss being mourned and requiring adjustment. Very extended periods of anticipatory grief may not be helpful, as 'grief work' involves emotional withdrawal from the love object. Such a process may not be suitable for the carer of a person with a chronic illness, as their loved one still requires care. In addition, a withdrawal of emotional involvement can be guilt-inducing.

Exercise

Talk to someone you know who has cared for a close relative or friend with a chronic disease (please ask their permission first and only proceed if they are willing). Make sure that you will not be interrupted. Ask them to recount their story (tape-record it if you are allowed to). Try to identify the transitions in their life, and losses/ gains that they have experienced. Ask them how they think about the future. You will need to be sensitive to their feelings. Remember that *listening* is a skill. Try not to interrupt or offer advice. If the person you are interviewing starts to cry, put a hand on theirs, or on their shoulder. Once they have stopped, ask them if they would prefer not to continue. Assuming that the interview reached a natural conclusion, how did this person seem at the end?

This type of exercise is helpful because it encourages health care professionals to listen and not to feel that they should give advice. It highlights one of the most important uses of non-directive counselling. This type of listening gives the person the opportunity to remember the individual as they were, recall happy and sad events and situations. They will often laugh as they recount happy occasions and cry as they remember sad ones. Most people prefer to continue with their story, if they are allowed to, once they have stopped crying. In recounting these events, they are able to find new meanings in them which can provide comfort and reassurance and hope for the future. People in these types of situation do not expect health professionals to provide solutions, but welcome support, empathy and the opportunity to talk. Most people appear to feel relieved and happier afterwards, provided the interview is not terminated abruptly.

Helping bereaved people

Nurses and other professional carers often have the difficult task of helping people immediately after the death of their loved one. Try to remember that these people may feel very shocked and numb. A lack of emotional expression does not mean they are alright. As it is often difficult to believe what has happened, especially if it is unexpected, it may be helpful for the relatives to see and – if they wish – touch the deceased person. Nurses can prepare the body by removing medical apparatus like intravenous infusions and drains and making sure the dead person is dressed in nightclothes and is covered with clean sheets. This is especially important after failed resuscitation attempts. It may be unhelpful for relatives to have a final memory which indicates suffering. Many people have not seen a dead body and are fearful of how a loved one might look. However, imagination may sometimes be worse than the real thing and mothers appear to adjust better if they have had the opportunity to hold their stillborn baby or dead child, no matter how damaged or deformed it appears to the staff. Nurses can help by initially remaining with them. Research indicates that relatives of very sick patients in intensive care units are often aware of the death or impending death of their loved one before biological (or brainstem) death is confirmed, yet they collude with medical and nursing staff in the pretence of recovery (Sque and Payne 1994).

When you give information to newly bereaved people, such as where to register the death, remember that concentration and memory may be poor. Use written information if possible. It is often helpful for relatives to have explicit instructions about how to deal with undertakers, wills and other arrangements. The majority of people cope with the experience of bereavement with help from their family and friends, and some may find support from bereavement support services like Cruse or Compassionate Friends or other services provided by palliative care units. Bereavement support is not necessarily required by all people, and may actually be unhelpful if it is forced on people, because it implies that they cannot cope (Payne and Relf 1994). However, it is good practice to routinely assess the bereavement follow-up needs of relatives. If we take a holistic view of clients and their families, care should not stop at the death of the client.

Summary

- Attachment is a reciprocal relationship that occurs as a result of long-term interactions.
- First attachments occur in infancy between the child and carer. They are characterized by mutual commitment and intense feelings.

- Separation produces the responses of protest, despair and emotional detachment.

- Attachment relationships are essential for adequate emotional, social and cognitive development.

- Loss of attachment objects is distressing.

- Grief occurs after all types of loss, but its intensity depends on the degree of attachment.

- Bereavement is a process experienced after the death or loss of an attachment object.

Further reading

Berk, L.E. (1991) *Child Development*, 2nd edn. Needhan Heights, MA: Allyn and Bacon. Chapter 10.

Haight, B.K. (1988) The therapeutic role of a structured life review process in homebound elderly subjects. *Journal of Gerontology: Psychological Sciences*, 43(2): 40–44.

Kennel, J.H., Voos, D.K. and Klaus, M.H. (1979) Parent–infant bonding. In J.D. Osofsky (ed.), *Handbook of Infant Development*. New York: John Wiley.

Littlewood, J. (1992) *Aspects of Grief*. London: Routledge.

Parry, G. (1990) *Coping with Crises*. Leicester: British Psychological Society/ Routledge.

PAIN

Introduction

We include this chapter because pain and other aspects of suffering are complex human problems which provide an opportunity to draw together many different psychological concepts and examine how psychology can make a valuable contribution to good nursing care. Case studies are provided and the reader is invited to consider how all of the psychological principles referred to in this book can contribute to understanding and dealing with the issues identified.

Very few people will not have experienced the unpleasant physical sensation of pain. The pain which accompanies traumas such as burns, cuts, strains or other injuries, represents a danger signal which prompts us to remove ourselves from a harmful situation and take action to treat or protect the injured area. In those rare conditions where the pain sensation is absent, the individual often dies from the results of repeated or extensive traumas or undiagnosed disease.

In considering the psychology of pain, the chapter will begin with children and work through the age range, referring *en route* to pain theories, common pain problems, pain assessment and psychological approaches to pain management.

Children: Feeling pain and learning to express pain

Some behavioural reactions to pain, such as withdrawal, wincing or crying out, appear to be reflex responses which even neonates exhibit. Midwives who have used the heel prick test for phenylketonuria will be well aware of the slight delay between the incision and the crying response as the pain signal is carried up the slow pain fibres to reach the brain and trigger a distress response. At one time it was assumed that preterm neonates did not have a nervous system which was capable of transmitting and registering pain. This belief has now been challenged as researchers have reported arousal responses to painful stimuli *in utero*.

Researchers and clinicians are now seriously concerned about the long-term effects of pain experienced by preterm neonates undergoing intensive care. There are strong indications that premature babies may later be more sensitive and less tolerant of pain. There are a number of possible explanations for this, which include a classically conditioned fear response, or the association of pain with unpleasant events which gives negative meaning to pain. Small babies are rarely, if ever, given analgesia or local anaesthesia for procedures in which this would be standard practice for an adult. Soothing interventions such as stroking the infant, or gently rubbing a post-incision site, can reduce pain and autonomic alarm responses, and provide comfort.

Responses to pain also involve voluntary behaviours which are learned throughout childhood, many of which are ways of communicating that we are in pain. Operant conditioning and modelling are two ways in which this is likely to occur. It is during this time that children learn how to cope, in different ways, with minor injuries and minor painful complaints.

Exercise

Think of ways in which adolescent boys and girls may be expected to differ in their responses to (1) pain due to physical trauma and (2) abdominal pain. Explain how these differences might have arisen and what influences this might have for ways of dealing with pain in adult life.

Different families treat pain in different ways and therefore individuals learn to cope with pain, and signal the presence of pain, in very different ways. For example, if a child is allowed to stay at home from school every time they complain of a tummy ache, it is little wonder that complaining of tummy ache becomes a useful way of avoiding unpleasant activities. In fact, many young children learn to complain of a headache or tummy ache without really understanding what it means, other than that it results in comfort and attention. This highlights the importance of learning processes in the shaping of pain responses. It also highlights some of the difficulties of assessing the causes of pain in young children. Even when children can verbalize their pain, their self-reports are based upon an understanding which may deviate from our own (see Chapter 3). It is not wise to take the location of the pain at face value, but to check by asking the child to point to it. Neither is it wise to use outward manifestations of pain, such as crying, as an accurate indicator of how bad the pain is in a small child.

Exercise

Think of reasons why a hospitalized 3-year-old in severe pain fails to complain of pain and remains quiet and withdrawn. How might you identify whether or not the child has pain and how bad the pain is?

Children who repeatedly use pain or discomfort as an avoidance strategy may fail to learn to cope adequately with stressful events, such as examinations or family squabbles. As adolescents, they may develop genuine stress-related tension headache or abdominal pain which continues the cycle of events into adulthood.

Children gradually learn to control their emotions and their behaviour as they grow older, and variations in response may become less obvious. However, there will remain individual variations in pain tolerance and pain expression. Health professionals may interpret these as differences in personality and, indeed, consistent patterns of response to painful situations and pain sensations do become part of an individual's psychological make-up and repertoire. Nevertheless, most people can benefit from learning new coping strategies for dealing with all sorts of painful situations.

Pain as a threat

Pain is an unpleasant sensation which accompanies a traumatic or disease process. However, those of you who have read *The Challenge of Pain* (Melzack and Wall 1988) will remember the painful initiation ceremonies which still take place in certain societies. Here, individuals do not express pain even in cases of deep penetration of the skin. Is this because it would bring disgrace to disclose pain? Or is it because the pain represents a challenge, rather than a threat? Or is it because the individuals are so excited that the pain sensation is suppressed?

Beecher (1959) is much quoted for his observations that soldiers frequently appeared to feel no pain as they were removed from the battlefield with terrible injuries. His interpretation was that this was a psychological phenomenon, attributable to relief at the prospect of reaching a safe environment. However, this is open to challenge. There are many examples of civilians who have experienced major trauma yet have felt no pain for a prolonged period after the injury. A better recent interpretation may be that the extreme state of arousal prompted by the need to reach safety suppresses the pain signal through the release of beta-endorphin. The absence of pain enables the individual to seek help or reach safety. One individual was reported to have carried his severed arm across several fields to obtain help after a farming accident. Only once safety is reached does the level of arousal subside and pain commence. This interpretation suggests that the phenomenon of post-traumatic analgesia may be due to a physiological survival mechanism, rather than a psychological process, although the two clearly interact with each other, since psychological appraisal stimulates physiological arousal (see Chapter 6). It is interesting to note that the reason distraction promotes pain control may also relate to the release of beta-endorphin, and not only to the diversion of attention.

Pain usually signals a threat to the body and may therefore be regarded as a stressor. Coping with pain is an important issue and the reader may wish to refer back to Chapter 6 to see how pain fits into the model of stress and coping proposed by Lazarus and Folkman (1984). The model helps to explain the relationship between acute pain and anxiety, since acute pain signals the presence of a stressor, while anxiety reflects the state of arousal which prompts coping actions. The individual's own appraisal of the situation, together with the perceived and actual personal or supportive resources available for coping with the painful event, are likely to determine their responses and outcomes. In line with the theory of locus of control (see Chapter 4), the individual may initiate personal action to deal with the pain, or seek help from others such as doctors, or do nothing and just hope that the pain will eventually go away. The ultimate failure to identify any way of dealing with persistent pain may result in feelings of helplessness, hopelessness and depression (similar to Selye's state of exhaustion or Seligman's 'learned helplessness').

The gate control theory of pain

It is now clear that physiological and psychological processes both contribute to the pain experience. However, it was not until the 1960s that Melzack and Wall formulated their gate control theory of pain to account for a wide variety of pain phenomena, including phantom limb pain. Ronald Melzack is a psychologist from McGill University, Canada and Patrick Wall a physiologist from London University. Their unique and formidable combination of knowledge and skills produced the first theory of pain which included descending pain control mechanisms which could modulate or inhibit ascending pain signals. This laid the theoretical basis for understanding that psychological influences on pain are not just 'all in the mind', but are directly capable of modifying pain sensations on their way to the brain. This theory gave credibility to psychological approaches to pain management, such as imagery and relaxation, and actually stimulated the development of pain treatments, such as transcutaneous electrical nerve stimulation (TENS).

Our current physiological understanding of the way the 'gate' operates is described elsewhere (see Carroll and Bowsher 1993: 11–14). The term 'gate' is purely a conceptual one used to describe a mechanism for pain inhibition. Inhibition may come about when the stimulation of peripheral A (large) nerve fibres overrides pain signals transmitted along C (small) nerve fibres. You may have noticed that when you automatically rub a painful area, it can actually have a powerful pain-reducing effect. In fact, TENS is based upon this principle.

As pain fibres enter the spinal cord, they may be subject to the inhibitory action of neurotransmitters such as the enkephalins (natural morphine-like substances). It is thought that acupuncture acts by releasing these chemical pain suppressants. Beta-endorphin, in addition to acting within the brain to suppress pain, circulates in the nervous system to act at a more local level. Beta-endorphin is under the control of the prefrontal lobe of the cerebral cortex, which is also associated with the emotions. Therefore, it is possible to see how psychological state may be directly associated with pain control. There is evidence that the cause-and-effect relationship between pain and psychological state may operate in both directions. Uncontrollable pain may trigger negative appraisals and negative emotions, leaving an individual feeling anxious or depressed. On the other hand, existing negative feelings may leave the pain gate open and make it more difficult for the individual to tolerate the resulting pain. This is why comprehensive assessment, together with an understanding about the ways in which pain mechanisms work, is necessary for patients when pain is difficult to control, particularly in chronic pain.

The placebo effect

The **placebo effect** is probably associated with the release of beta-endorphin, triggered by psychological expectation. This effect can be very powerful (equivalent to a small therapeutic dose of morphine). It therefore tends to confound studies designed to evaluate the effectiveness of any analgesic drug. This is why all drug trials take the form of a **randomized controlled trial** (RCT), which compares the effects of the drug against a similar looking dummy which contains no active ingredient – that is, a placebo. The research design (the double-blind procedure) also ensures that those who administer the medication cannot signal their awareness of the content and influence patient expectations (see non-verbal communication in Chapter 9).

If the administration of a **placebo** results in the elimination or reduction of the patient's pain, this does *not* indicate that the pain was not real at all but existed only in the mind. The release of natural endorphin through this process is capable of helping to control all types of pain. However, it should be noted that not all people are responsive in this way.

Health care professionals can make therapeutic use of the placebo effect to boost the effect of analgesic drugs and other treatments by encouraging patients to have confidence in the treatment they are receiving. However, it is worth remembering that unrealistic expectations may damage future relationships and wipe out any subsequent placebo effects. Furthermore, even when there is a good placebo effect, it tends to diminish with subsequent doses as the body becomes aware that it is receiving no active ingredient. It is therefore not a suitable substitute for real analgesia and is unlikely to sustain long-term effects for people with chronic pain.

Defining acute and chronic pain

Acute pain has been differentiated from chronic pain on the basis of duration. However, this is no longer felt to be a useful classification. The main differentiation, from a psychological perspective, relates to the cognitive and behavioural processes of adaptation which take place when someone experiences persistent pain. The way that someone views the meaning of pain during an acute episode which is believed to be self-limiting, is likely to be quite different from the way they feel and react to an undiagnosed pain which shows no sign of ever going away and fails to respond to treatment. The time taken to realize that the pain is showing no signs of remitting is a function of the individual's beliefs and of the physiological cause of the pain (see Waddell 1992), both of which are subject to wide variations.

Some types of pain, such as migraine or angina, involve recurrent acute episodes. Some individuals respond to, and manage, each attack as an acute episode but remain fully functional in between. Others find that their lives are completely disrupted by the constant threat of a repeated attack and become chronic pain sufferers. Much depends on the personal and supportive resources they have available to cope with what are very unpleasant and potentially frightening symptoms.

Pain in malignant disease is another example of pain which does not conveniently fit into either category and will be considered further below. It is important to remember that the individual interpretation and response is much more important than any arbitrary textbook definition, when making an assessment or identifying suitable approaches to treatment.

Acute pain

Acute pain may be related to trauma or disease. It prompts personal action and help-seeking. It is one of the main symptoms which causes individuals to visit their doctor. Acute pain may also result from invasive techniques conducted as part of medical investigations, surgery or treatments. All health professionals owe a duty of care to patients to minimize the infliction of pain and assist in reducing the intensity of acute pain if the individual finds it difficult to tolerate. As such, the administration of analgesia is an important part of acute pain control, as are psychological methods of pain control. The latter are considered below.

Preparation for painful procedures

The importance of preparation for all planned procedures, particularly those which might result in pain, has long been recognized, and was referred to in Chapter 6. It has been clearly demonstrated that pre-operative information-giving results in a reduction of anxiety and post-operative pain (for examples, see Hayward 1974; Boore 1978; Seers 1989).

The Lazarus theory of stress and coping provides an understanding of how this process occurs and what type of information is likely to be beneficial. First, information about what is going to happen before, during and after the procedure increases arousal and helps the individual to prepare themselves for what is to come. This should include information about the pain and other sensations which the individual is likely to experience. This type of information reduces stress through the reduction of uncertainty and unpredictability (see Chapter 6). There is *no* evidence that this is likely to induce pain through the self-fulfilling prophecy. Rather, the reverse is true – because people are less frightened, they tend to report less pain.

Second, and as important, is information about what individuals can do to help themselves when they have pain. This information is designed to assist in the coping process and enhance the level of personal control experienced by the patient. It is useful to find out what stress management skills the individual already has, or prefers to use, and encourage their use. Useful strategies include controlled breathing, relaxation, distraction and imagery (see McCaffery and Beebe 1994). Patients who have not used these before may need some assistance and encouragement. It is not easy to relax when you don't know how, particularly when you have pain. In fact, ante-natal classes provide a good example of preventive education in pain control. It may not be feasible to provide group instruction for surgical patients, but it should be possible to send some basic instructional literature to those on the waiting list.

Third, it is important for patients to feel that support is available when they are experiencing pain. Patients need to have an alarm bell handy and be encouraged to use it when necessary. They also need to know what help is available in terms of analgesia and be encouraged to take full advantage of it.

Early discharge increasingly means that patients are sent home before post-operative pain is properly under control. Patients must be given appropriate medication to take home with them. They need to know what to expect in terms of pain and when to summon medical help.

Administration of analgesic drugs in acute pain

There is a big difference between managing our own pain and managing someone else's pain. One of the key issues is that of perceived control.

Research has demonstrated that individuals will put up with far more pain if they know they can control it if they want to, than if they have no control. Promoting personal control over pain is an important issue for health care professionals working in areas where it is they, rather than the patient, who exercises control.

Case study: Mary

Mary gets frequent headaches which have occasionally developed into a full migraine (blinding headache and vomiting). However, she has found that she can usually control them by taking a particular OTC (over-the-counter) analgesic at an early stage. She is admitted to hospital for routine surgery. Her tablets have been taken away from her. She develops a headache which gets worse as her anxiety increases. She sees the drug round taking place and asks the staff for her tablets. They refuse to let her have them, but offer to get a substitute drug written up by the doctor when he comes round later.

Exercise

Put yourself in Mary's position. How do you think that she thinks and feels? What is her response likely to be? Put yourself in the position of the staff. What are they likely to be thinking? What can they do about it? Now consider the advantages and disadvantages of self-medication in hospital.

Patient-controlled analgesia

Research into the relationship between personal control and pain intensity led directly to the introduction of patient-controlled analgesia (PCA) for the control of post-operative pain and pain in malignancy. A number of studies have consistently demonstrated that most (though not all) post-operative patients report better pain control when they have PCA than when analgesia is administered by nurses (Owen *et al*. 1991).

Patient-controlled analgesia has been used successfully with children (see Berde 1991) and the elderly, although there is a tendency to limit its use with these groups. There are, however, some words of caution about the use of PCA. The reader who is now familiar with the concept of locus of control might predict that people with internal locus of control would have a greater preference for PCA than those with external locus of control. This issue is not yet fully researched and is worthy of further investigation. It is certainly necessary to promote personal control by ensuring that all patients are fully familiar with how to use the apparatus. Some may require further assistance to get the hang of using it, particularly in the early stages of recovery or when the pain is so severe that their sense of self-efficacy is reduced. Patients often need to be encouraged to administer a dose prior to movement or physiotherapy in order to facilitate their recovery.

Case study: Sarah

An elderly woman, Sarah, is given PCA immediately following a hip replacement. She is later seen to be restless and appears to be in great pain. Inspection reveals that she is not using the apparatus. The nurse is heard talking to Sarah as though speaking to a small child. The nurse tells Sarah she must remember to press the little button when she is in pain and shows her where it is.

Exercise

Is the nurse's action appropriate and, if not, why not? What should the nurse do to ensure that Sarah's pain is maintained under proper control? What are the possible consequences if the pain is not properly controlled?

There is now a large body of research evidence which demonstrates that hospital staff underestimate pain intensity and tend to under medicate (Seers and Davis 1993). This applies to all age groups, but in particular to children and the elderly. There is no evidence that the elderly feel less pain than other age groups, but they tend to complain less because they don't like to make a fuss, and tolerate more pain because they have had more experience of coping with it during their lifetime. This is why routine pain assessment is so important to determine actual levels of pain and suffering.

Assessing acute pain

The assessment of acute pain centres upon the use of simple scales to identify pain intensity (no pain to worst pain imaginable), pain tolerance (no pain to totally unbearable pain) and responses to treatment in terms of pain relief (complete relief to no relief at all). Scales need to take into account any visual or hearing loss, and the level of understanding of the individual being assessed. The details of assessment scales can be found elsewhere (see, e.g. Carroll and Bowsher 1993).

Visual analogue scales are useful for research purposes because they provide interval data, but are best presented vertically, as shown in Fig.

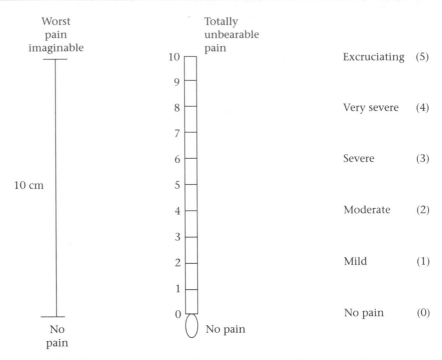

Figure 8.1 Visual analogue, pain thermometer and verbal rating scales.

8.1. Graduation marks (no more than 10) are sometimes added for clinical purposes to form a pain thermometer. The one illustrated is adapted from Hayward (1974). Five- or six-point verbal rating scales are usually adequate for clinical use with the normal adult and elderly populations. Verbal presentation will be needed for those with visual limitations, including those who have not got their glasses on! In fact, those presented in Fig. 8.1 can be used in any combination which appear most suitable for a particular group of patients.

Happy–sad faces scales (see Fig. 8.2) are useful for young children, those with learning difficulties and the confused elderly, provided they have adequate vision. Please ensure that those who need glasses to see this are wearing them! This scale probably reflects bearability, rather than actual pain intensity.

The aim of acute pain management

It is difficult to find a level of pain intensity which may be regarded as acceptable for everyone. Therefore, a useful aim for the management of acute pain is: 'The patient should never have more pain than he or she can willingly bear'.

Although there is a close relationship between pain intensity and bearability in most instances, there will be variations in pain tolerance and perceived pain control which can widen the gap. The assessment of

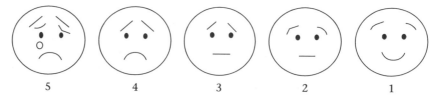

Figure 8.2 A happy/sad faces scale of pain intensity/bearability.

pain intensity together with pain bearability should help to ensure that the patient is receiving the help that is needed. Some patients may need to be discouraged from pushing themselves to the limits of their endurance, while others may genuinely be able to tolerate high levels of pain intensity without undue suffering.

One of the main reasons for the regular assessment of pain using these measures is that patients are frequently unwilling to draw attention to the presence of pain for fear of appearing a wimp or because they don't want to trouble the busy nurse. Routine assessment is also a way of communication with other medical and health care professionals so that the patient receives sufficient analgesia (see Sofaer 1993) and so that complications which may be contributing to the pain can be identified. Sofaer (1985) and Miaskowski (1994) have highlighted the importance of good interpersonal care in determining effective pain control, patient satisfaction and patient outcomes.

Pain is what the person says it is and exists whenever they say it does

The absence of an obvious cause does not imply that the pain is not real, although there is evidence that nursing students react less favourably to patients who do not have a firm diagnosis (Gillmore and Hill 1981). Medical technology has not yet advanced to the stage of being able to diagnose all causes of pain. We have no way of knowing if the patient's pain gating mechanism is open or closed. If we make assumptions about the patient's pain, regardless of their complaints, we may turn out to be completely wrong.

Case study: Sue

Sue is the mother of two mentally handicapped children aged 8 and 10 years, respectively, who require total physical care. She developed severe carpal tunnel syndrome in both hands and eventually had surgery to her right (dominant) hand. Her post-operative complaints of pain extending up to her shoulder were dismissed: 'Your operation was on your hand, not your shoulder'. She was discharged on the third day (a Friday) with no analgesia. By the time she got home the pain was unbearable. Over-the-counter analgesics had no effect and she borrowed some Distalgesic tablets from a friend to tide her over the weekend until she could visit her GP. She went to the pain clinic some months later where she was diagnosed as having sympathetic reflex dystrophy. This is a post-traumatic complication (fortunately not too common) which gives rise to severe pain radiating from the site of the original injury. Sue was distressed that the possibility of such a complication had not been pointed out to her before the operation, as she was now much worse off than she had been before. However, this was not the main source of her present anger.

Exercise

Consider why staff might have dismissed or minimized Sue's complaints of pain prior to discharge. Why do you think that Sue is still upset about her treatment? What could the staff have done to reduce her distress and continued suffering?

Now put yourself in Sue's position three years into the future. You have recently had a lot of problems and are advised to have a hysterectomy. How would you feel about this? You have little choice and decide to proceed. What do think your attitudes towards the medical, nursing and other health care staff are likely to be? How do you think they might help to reassure you in the pre-operative and post-operative situation?

Chronic pain

Exercise

Imagine that you wake up one morning with a severe pain in your lower back after helping to lift a heavy patient from an awkward position the day before. What are your thoughts? What do you do? You see the doctor who tells you to go and lie flat and take regular analgesics, but it feels even worse after 2 weeks. What are your thoughts? You go back to the doctor who thinks that you may have a trapped nerve and refers you to an orthopaedic consultant which will involve a 6-week wait. What do you do in the meantime and why?

Interviews with patients attending pain clinics with low back pain indicate that this is a common scenario. Sadly, some of these patients are still waiting for a positive diagnosis and spend most of their lives lying down, even after 10 years. Most back pain, particularly where onset is delayed after the likely causal incident, is actually caused by muscle strain and subsequent inflammation. People with symptoms such as those above should never be advised to rest for more than 2 days unless medical examination indicates nerve involvement or the possibility of bony metastases. Otherwise, individuals should be referred to a physiotherapist for immediate advice and exercises to maintain posture and mobility.

Bed rest quickly reduces muscle tone and thereby increases pain on movement. Prolonged bed rest following a back injury can result in painful muscle spasms, which lead the individual to believe that any movement is causing further damage to 'trapped nerves' in their back. A vicious cycle is established in which the individual does less, loses fitness, loses their job, and increasingly allows others to undertake self-care tasks for them. These problems have been described by Waddell (1992) as iatrogenic (caused by medical advice) consequences of prolonged bed rest. Quality of life is destroyed, resulting in psychological distress and even depression. This psychological state leaves the pain gate open and results in even more pain, exacerbated by spasm and tension in the individual's weakened muscles. Other life stressors serve to make the situation worse by increasing anxiety and tension, and are themselves more difficult to cope with because of the pain, loss of concentration, decreased mobility and increased distress. Behavioural responses will depend upon the availability of personal and supportive resources. These may be adaptive and make the situation better or be maladaptive and make the situation worse. Some of the factors which influence these outcomes are considered below.

Chronic pain, whatever the cause, may be extremely difficult, if not impossible, to eliminate. Chronic pain is often associated with depression. However, the debate among pain researchers about whether depression causes pain or chronic pain causes depression is really somewhat irrelevant if the relationship is viewed as a dynamic cycle. Pain is rarely, if ever, the sole cause of depression. Helping an individual to cope with other problems in their lives may be as important as helping them to reduce their pain. A full assessment should include a range of potential stressors and coping resources which require attention. Some of these are reviewed below.

Information

Patients who have persistent pain need the opportunity to discuss the causes and potential consequences of their condition and to understand what is causing or contributing to the pain. Many fear, quite wrongly, that they have a serious condition, such as cancer, or that their pain and disability will get progressively worse. Few will actually admit to this unless given some encouragement in a relaxed and friendly environment; however, such fears can only be allayed once they have been expressed.

Case study: Margaret

Margaret, a middle-aged lady, attended the pain clinic with a mild to moderate pain below the right shoulder blade. An initial interview revealed that she had had this pain for several years and found it extremely intrusive in her life. It gradually emerged that a friend of her's had died of breast cancer in a lot of pain and she was afraid that the same thing was happening to her. It had taken a long time for her to pluck up the courage to report the pain to her doctor, though she had not voiced her fears. A thorough medical examination in the clinic, including breast examination and X-rays, revealed nothing. However, a numb area of skin in the painful region indicated that she was probably suffering from post-herpetic neuralgia. The doctor took some time to explain this to her in detail, and to offer TENS as a possible treatment to help relieve the pain if it still troubled her at the next visit.

It would have been easy to label Margaret as being 'neurotic' and to dismiss her pain as insignificant. However, it was a very different woman that returned a few weeks later, full of smiles, who said that her life had been 'transformed'. After years of suffering and worry, the gate seemed to have closed and she was now hardly aware that the pain was still there.

The above case study illustrates the potential importance of information about the diagnosis and prognosis. Many people with chronic pain who do not have a diagnosis have said that they would actually prefer to know that they had cancer so that they knew what they were dealing with. Some people have expressed relief on being told that they have multiple sclerosis because they now know that the pain is real and they are not going mad.

Increasing levels of activity and involvement

Many patients with chronic pain have disengaged themselves from previous occupational and social activities. The case of Pam, the smoker with Raynaud's disease in Chapter 4, is a good example of this. This leaves them with little to do and little to distract themselves from the pain, thus creating another vicious cycle. Fordyce (1976) introduced operant behavioural treatments for chronic pain patients, particularly those with back pain. This approach means that significant others must learn to ignore verbal and non-verbal pain behaviours and complaints, while responding positively to activities which are initiated by the pain patient. It has been used successfully to increase adaptive behaviours and decrease maladaptive (usually avoidance) behaviours. It has been shown to lead to a reduction in medication consumption and depression (Linton 1985). For this reason, the physiotherapist and occupational therapist are important members of the multidisciplinary pain team. Patients ideally need a programme of activity and increasing physical exercise tailored to suit their individual requirements. It is not easy for them to undertake what amounts to major life changes and they may require a lot of reassurance and encouragement.

Hobbies and social commitments are important sources of distraction and involvement. In fact, any increase in activity and involvement increases quality of life for chronic pain patients, even when the intensity and frequency of the pain remains the same. Involvement in household chores is an important source of activity for most people. It can be very difficult for significant others to restrain themselves from stepping in to help someone in pain. Not only is it seen as humane to help, but it can be much quicker to do things themselves. This is why it has been shown that patients with more solicitous spouses experience more pain and depression and less activity (see Chapter 4). It is also worth remembering that increased mobility can have financially damaging implications for those in receipt of state disability benefits. This is one of the reasons it may be difficult to persuade people who have become chronic invalids to attempt to walk out in the street, attend the gym or go swimming.

It is common for people who feel better to engage in a sudden burst of activity, often pushing themselves to their limit. They pay for this later through increased pain. This confirms their belief that exercise or movement is harming them and leads to further avoidance of activity. Chronic pain patients need to learn to 'pace themselves' so that they keep to a regular and increasing schedule of activity and exercise. Maladaptive behaviours, such as avoidance of anything which is thought likely to cause pain, are learned from an early stage in the development of the painful condition. Overall, there needs to be a better understanding in primary health care of chronic pain processes and greater emphasis on prevention and immediate and continuing rehabilitation for people with chronic painful conditions in order to prevent them from becoming incapacitated by maladaptive responses in the first place.

The impact of past and present experiences and stressors

Our past experiences shape our beliefs about, and attitudes towards, a whole range of present events and situations. It is not just past experiences of pain which shape future responses to pain, but past experiences of coping with all types of stressful or difficult situations. Thus some people are better equipped with coping strategies to deal with a chronic painful condition than others. Those who cope well with chronic pain are probably in the majority. It is the minority who fail to cope or who cope poorly that attract the attention of health care professionals in pain clinics. These patients normally comprise the sample in chronic pain research and it is important to recognise that they are not necessarily representative of chronic pain patients in general. Poor coping in some of these patients may be what has led some observers to refer to 'the pain-prone patient' (Engel 1959) and to seek psychoanalytic or personality trait explanations. However, Sternbach and Timmermans (1975) found that chronic back pain patients who responded successfully to surgery showed significant reductions in measures of neuroticism and hypochondriasis, indicating that these are more likely to be a result of chronic pain rather than the cause, and are therefore reversible.

Walker *et al.* (1990) found that older people with chronic pain are more likely to experience psychological distress if they are dissatisfied with their past lives or are experiencing current stressors, such as personal relationship problems. This is in keeping with Erikson's final life transition to a state of integrity or despair (see Chapter 7). Once again, it is difficult to establish cause and effect. Chronic pain affects all aspects of life (see Roy 1992). It disrupts 'normal' lifestyle, changes expectations, and requires substantial adjustments. Some find this easier than others, but those who find it hardest to accept appear to be those who feel that life in general has been unfair to them. These people are often bitter, alienated, complaining and depressed. Their negativity may leave the pain gate wide open. They are hardest for health professionals to help, but they deserve and need genuine concern, understanding and time before any educational and activity programme can be encouraged. Treatments which take into account a variety of these issues are outlined in Holzman and Turk (1986).

Chronic pain places huge strains on family and interpersonal relationships (Snelling 1994). Roy (1992) has noted that family therapy may be beneficial for chronic pain patients in order to help both parties in the relationship to come to terms with the painful condition and to help them to cope effectively. Very often, pain is blamed for the breakdown of a relationship, whereas in reality the relationship may have been frail from the outset. Addressing family strains or breakdown at the same time as treating the pain is likely to be more successful than trying to treat pain in isolation from the situation in which it is experienced.

The availability of personal pain-controlling strategies

Many people who have chronic pain learn to develop active coping strategies which help them to keep their pain under control. Depending upon the type of pain and the age of the patient, these include such simple expedients as ensuring that clothing and footwear are comfortable, provide warmth (body warmers are very useful) and are easy to put on and take off (Velcro-fastened trainers are useful); finding a comfortable chair which provides good upright support; situating a commode near the bed for night time use; allowing plenty of time to get up in the morning; doing regular gentle exercises to keep muscles and joints toned; avoiding foods which might precipitate pain; using preparatory pain-relieving sprays, ointments, creams or other home remedies; using TENS; applying heat through hot water bottles or heated pads; using methods of distraction and keeping occupied. Walker *et al.* (1990) found that the more pain-controlling strategies older people used, the better their pain control and the less distressed they were.

A number of studies (e.g. Brown and Nicassio 1987) have demonstrated that chronic pain patients who use active coping strategies and have internal locus of control are less depressed than those with external locus of control who use passive coping strategies (hoping or praying) or relying on others for treatment of pain. Harkapaa *et al.* (1991) demonstrated that those with internal beliefs had better treatment outcomes and were more likely to persevere with exercises during a 3-month follow-up period. All chronic pain sufferers should be encouraged to search for and recognize strategies which suit them and which they are motivated to use themselves on a regular basis. Advice from a physiotherapist and occupational therapist can be valuable in identifying new techniques and strategies for daily living.

Assessing and treating chronic pain

The assessment of pain intensity is only a small part of the assessment of chronic pain, alongside the above issues. It is useful to use a simple verbal rating scale to identify how bad the pain is when it is at its worst so that precipitating factors can be identified. It is also useful to know how bad the pain is when it is least troublesome. In other words, is the patient ever pain-free and, if so, under what circumstances? A pain diary may be useful to record these details over a 1-week period in order to expose triggering and minimizing factors which are not otherwise obvious. This is a type of functional analysis, which was referred to in Chapter 4.

It is essential to identify what the patient thinks might be causing the pain and to ensure that a thorough explanation is offered following a thorough investigation. An explanation of the way the pain gate works, and the effects of other stressors and personal feelings, should be given. This will ensure that the patient understands that there is no suggestion that the pain is not real, but that therapy depends upon the treatment of the whole person and not just the painful part.

Explanations for the rationale for each treatment need to be given and patients should be involved in deciding which therapeutic approach is best for them. The case study below illustrates how misconceptions can lead to unnecessary treatments.

Case study: Harry

A young man called Harry came to the pain clinic with ankylosing spondylitis. He already had a good understanding of the cause of his pain and found regular exercise to be his most beneficial personal coping strategy. He was actually coping very well. However, he was keen to explore all avenues in terms of possible treatments and had heard about the benefits of acupuncture. The doctor agreed to commence a course and while the needles were being inserted he was asked what he expected of acupuncture. Harry explained that he believed that acupuncture would disentangle the nerves in his back and that this would cure his pain. After the doctor had explained to him how acupuncture actually worked and what effects could be expected, he decided not to continue with the course of treatment.

Multidisciplinary pain programmes which include cognitive–behavioural treatments have been evaluated as being successful for chronic pain patients. For example, St. Thomas' Hospital, London has been running a successful in-patient programme for a number of years (Williams *et al.* 1993). Depending upon initial and continuing assessments, psychological approaches to the treatment of chronic pain may include the following:

- Educate the patient about the gate control theory of pain and its implications.
- Provide information and explanations about the painful condition which are tailored to meet individual needs.
- Encourage the short-term use of a diary to identify avoidable pain-triggering factors and desirable pain-reducing factors.
- Initiate and teach behavioural approaches to increase activity and exercise and decrease dependence.
- Involve significant others in increasing the patient's independence.
- Offer counselling or life review to help individuals come to terms with events of the past and their present situation.
- Offer family therapy to rebuild relationships and secure social support networks.
- Offer training in relaxation and stress management techniques to control tension and anxiety and increase personal control over pain.
- Train individuals in the use of TENS, where appropriate, to close the pain gate peripherally and increase personal control over pain.
- Encourage individuals to develop as many strategies as they can to gain control over their own pain.
- Anti-depressants may be used in small doses (from as little as 10 mg of amitryptilline) at night to facilitate rest and control over continuous pain.
- Encourage the taking of effective analgesics for short periods to control exacerbations of pain and offer limited respite from continuous pain, thereby increasing perceived controllability.

The role of drugs in chronic pain

Over-the-counter or mild analgesics often have little impact on chronic pain and it is tempting to resort to the prescription of stronger analgesics. One of the problems is that tolerance to analgesics tends to increase over time and leads to increasing dosages and the administration of stronger analgesics. The role of restricted analgesic drugs, such as morphine sulphate tablets (MST), in the control of chronic pain is contentious because of this effect and most pain clinics try to wean patients off regular long-term use of these types of drug. It is also necessary to recognize the competing roles of agonists and antagonists (see McCaffery and Beebe 1994), since they may end up cancelling each other out.

Analgesics are normally prescribed according to a regular time schedule which may not meet the patient's needs at all. The assessment of triggering factors should identify situations when the pain is increased, for example when getting up in the morning in the case of arthritis. It is therefore sensible to take analgesics in advance of activities or events which are likely to trigger pain, and not at other times. In this respect, the management of chronic pain is entirely different from the management of acute pain or pain in terminal illness. The patient should become their own therapist and take the most suitable drug only when it is necessary. Increasing dosages should act as a warning sign to seek further help.

Much time is spent in chronic pain clinics weaning people off analgesic drugs to which they have become tolerant. The reasons why their pain is uncontrollable often lies in some of the psychosocial issues identified above, although these are likely to be overlooked if a medical model of pain is applied.

Anti-depressant drugs have been found, in small dosages, to have a direct pain-controlling and relaxing effect and can be used therapeutically in pain patients who are not depressed, for example in neurogenic pain which is continuous. The dosage used is much smaller than that commonly used to treat depression and is usually taken at night to aid sleep.

Anxiolytics play no part in the treatment of chronic pain and can cause addiction. Where tension and muscle spasm are contributory factors in the pain, the initiation of a suitable exercise and activity programme, together with relaxation, stress management and attention to the factors identified above, offer a better approach to treatment.

The chronic pain patient in hospital

The most common cause of persistent pain in the general population is some type of arthritis. Therefore, the increasing age of the hospitalized population ensures that more and more people who are admitted for medical or surgical treatment will also have chronic pain. The needs of this group are extremely neglected, particularly when the focus of their hospital treatment is on a condition other than the one which gives rise to their pain. Their pain will inevitably be worse in hospital because they no longer have access to the personal coping strategies which they have developed at home. For example, some elderly people are able to remember the height of the bed and every obstacle they met on the way to the toilet, months after being in hospital. People in pain become very irritable with those around them. Nothing is more likely to provoke anger than any attempt to move an arthritis patient without first saying what you need to do and negotiating the best way of achieving this. As one patient commented after a nurse had tried to move her leg hurriedly, 'You lose control with the unexpected'.

Routine assessment on admission should include chronic pain and the means by which it is usually controlled. The availability of self-medication, the use of a commode at night, the offer of a hot water bottle, etc., should then be tailored to suit individual needs. This will reduce much distress and will save a lot of time in the long run. Advice from a physiotherapist or occupational therapist may be useful to assist a chronic pain patient to develop useful ways of coping while in hospital.

Pain in terminal illness

Malignant disease can give rise to severe pain over a prolonged period and this can, in some instances, be very difficult to treat. Assessment and treatment needs to combine the best principles of acute and chronic pain management.

The assessment of pain and administration of analgesia in intractable pain caused by malignant disease should be identical to the approach used in acute pain. Dosages of analgesia, whether administered by self or others, should be carefully titrated to suit individual needs and ensure that the pain never exceeds the ability of the patient to bear it. It is essential to ensure that the drugs used do not exert competing effects (see McCaffery and Beebe 1994). Regular assessment should ensure that the patient's pain is maintained within tolerable limits. This may require very large doses of analgesia. However, it is essential that drug-induced side-effects, such as nausea, are controlled along with the pain, as some people find these more intolerable than pain. Some people prefer to put up with pain, rather than feel that the drugs are making them lose control over what is going on. Assessment and care of the terminally ill patient should take into account all aspects of their current concerns and focus upon meeting all of their needs, not just the pain.

Case study: Mrs L.

Mrs L. was a 92-year-old lady who had lived alone for many years and was fiercely independent. A friend who had not seen her for some time called by chance to find that she was now bed-bound with abdominal cancer and was about to be forcibly admitted to the local hospice. The doctors arranging this were heard to say 'she must be in terrible pain'. Before the ambulance arrived, Mrs L. gleefully showed the friend the Diconal tablets she had hidden under her pillow. She knew she had cancer, but seemed to regard this as a relatively small challenge in comparison with the suffering she had endured during her long and hard life. The friend saw her shortly after admission, sitting up in bed complaining vigorously about having been bathed, but obviously enjoying the attention and triumphantly ordering sherry from the trolley. Just after this, the nurse came and gave her an injection with no attempt at an explanation, perhaps because she was profoundly deaf. This was the last time the friend was able to talk to her, as she lapsed into unconsciousness and died shortly after.

Exercise

Who should decide how much pain an individual has, and what treatment they should have? How can this be assessed and negotiated with someone who is profoundly deaf?

Information-giving is an important component of pain control in malignant disease. However, while most people prefer to know what is wrong with them so they can cope in their own way, there are a small number of individuals, possibly those with external (chance) locus of control, who prefer not to know and are unable to cope if the knowledge is forced upon them. It is probably preferable to ask people how much they wish to be told. Some people are very candid about it saying, if asked, 'I really don't want to know'.

Case study: Amy

Amy was a mother of four young children in her mid-thirties who had developed cervical cancer. She had recently experienced financial, housing and marital problems which had caused a lot of anxiety. Her distress increased as her symptoms became more obvious and the pain worsened. The health visitor and social worker asked the doctor to tell her about her condition, but he refused and said that she would be unable to cope with it. Eventually, her husband told her and her relief was evident to everyone. Once it was in the open, she was referred to the local hospice for care and pain control. Amy was able to make plans with the help of a social worker for the future of her children. She enjoyed her favourite hobby, painting, which distracted her from her other problems. She died a few weeks later with her pain well controlled and appearing happier than she had been for a long time.

Exercise

Why was the doctor reluctant to tell Amy what was wrong? Which model of anxiety do you think he was using? What would you have done if you had been the health visitor in this situation, and how would you have felt?

Health professionals frequently find it hard to discuss death and dying with patients because their own feelings about death, their sorrow at the prospect of losing someone they are getting close to, and inability to cope with the distress they predict it will precipitate, all get in the way. However, nothing is guaranteed to reduce pain control more than the uncertainty associated with not knowing what the cause of the pain is. Pain intensity interacts with perceived threat to determine pain tolerance. Not knowing what the cause of a pain is makes it impossible to cope with it. As soon as a positive diagnosis has been made, the health professional should discuss with the patient what their information needs are and how much they wish to be told. Those who cannot cope with being told the truth may use denial as a defence mechanism, or they may cling to the hope of a miracle. There is hope to be found in every situation, whether in the possibility of a miracle, or in meeting a loved one after death, or in celebrating past achievements or happinesses. Death is an inevitable, but not a hopeless, state. Uncontrollable pain is associated with hopelessness, not death, and a positive attitude will foster good pain control. Giving time and encouragement to talk with a sympathetic listener can be a great relief, and greatly enhance the pain-controlling effects of medical therapies.

The control of other unpleasant symptoms

There are many unpleasant symptoms which may be as difficult to cope with as pain – for example, nausea, vomiting, breathlessness and skin irritation. There is no reason why the principles of psychological management for these should be any different from those which are applied in pain management. The case study offered below uses the example of persistent itch. It highlights the importance of self-control and self-medication for people with chronic conditions.

Case study: William

William, an elderly gentleman who, for years, had suffered from psoriasis, was admitted to hospital following a stroke which caused a left-sided hemiplegia (he was right-handed). Fortunately, he soon started to recover function on the affected side and then asked for his own Betnovate ointment so that he could treat his psoriasis. The nurse insisted that he could only have it when she brought the drug trolley round. The itch now became a major preoccupation which led to increased irritability and angry outbursts directed at the over-stretched staff. Following his request to speak to the manager, his ointment was returned to him. This restored his sense of personal control and his emotional control, and the irritation ceased to be a source of complaint.

Exercise

Consider the potential merits of self-medication for elderly people in hospital. Now weigh these against the potential problems. What are the important issues for a hospital policy on self-medication in the elderly?

Summary

- Babies experience pain from the time they are born, but learn the meaning of pain and how to express it or suppress it as they grow older.

- Pain is a biopsychosocial phenomenon in which psychological factors interact with physiological factors at all levels to produce the pain experience.

- Preparation for painful procedures improves pain control.

- Personal control increases pain tolerance for all types of pain.

- Pain intensity and bearability can be assessed using simple self-report scales.

- Chronic pain is multifactorial and affects every aspect of life.

- Chronic pain requires multifactorial assessment and treatment.

- Cognitive-behavioural treatments for chronic pain aim to increase activity and reduce dependence and depression.

- Pain control in terminal illness should take account of all aspects of the patients' concerns, as well as the severity of their pain, since these interact to influence pain tolerance.

- Coping principles, including those of encouraging personal coping strategies, are important in controlling all types of unpleasant symptoms.

Further reading

Carroll, D. and Bowsher, D. (eds) (1993) *Pain: Management and Nursing Care*. Oxford: Butterworth-Heinemann.

Hayward, J.A. (1974) *Information – A Prescription Against Pain*. London: Scutari.

Holzman, A.D. and Turk, D.C. (1986) *Pain Management: A Handbook of Psychological Treatment Approaches*. New York: Pergamon Press.

McCaffery, M. and Beebe, A. (eds) (1994) *Pain: Clinical Manual for Nursing Practice*. London: C.V. Mosby.

SOCIAL PROCESSES IN HEALTH CARE DELIVERY

Introduction

This chapter focuses upon the effects of social influence on a number of different social aspects of health care, using theory and research from social psychology. First, we explore issues of relevance to health education and promotion, notably attitude change and persuasion. Then, we look at the importance of non-verbal behaviour in social interaction. Finally, we examine issues related to organizational processes in the delivery of health care.

Attitudes and attitude change

Attitudes and attitude change are central to the **social cognition** models of human behaviour, particularly the theory of planned behaviour, which were outlined in Chapter 2. Research and theory about attitudes are included within social psychology because, although they refer to private and subjective thought processes, they are formed by social influences and shape the ways that we behave towards other people.

Attitudes are evaluative subjective experiences which relate to some issue or object and involve judgement. They have assumed great importance within social psychology and health psychology. Attitude surveys are used by marketing firms to test public acceptance of new products, and by health promoters to test public reactions to mass campaigns. The assumption underlying these is that attitudes predispose the individual to respond or behave in a certain way.

Attitudes are generally conceptualized as consisting of three classes of response:

- affective (evaluative feelings)
- behavioural (overt actions)
- cognitive (opinions and beliefs)

These are commonly assessed using self-report measures, for example a series of statements accompanied by a Likert scale of agreement/disagreement, as illustrated by the example given in Fig. 9.1. Agreement/disagreement can be measured using an **ordinal** scale, as indicated, and these scores can be used for research or audit purposes.

It is usually the case that the three components of attitudes are congruent, and that the behavioural component of an attitude refers to the behaviour which is the object of that attitude. For example, if an individual approves of eating wholemeal bread, they are likely to eat wholemeal bread. However, the cause-and-effect relationship between these affective and behavioural components is not necessarily straightforward. An individual may begin to approve of a behaviour only after they have started to engage in it. For

Statement	Strongly agree	Agree	Uncertain/ don't know/ no opinion	Disagree	Strongly disagree
	5	4	3	2	1
I like playing squash		√			

Figure 9.1 Illustration of the measurement of a positive attitude towards playing squash, using a 5-point Likert scale.

example, a couple started eating wholemeal bread when they had visitors whom they knew would not approve of eating white bread. In other words, they responded to perceived **normative** pressure (social influence), even though they did not particularly want to change. Only as they continued to eat wholemeal bread did they develop a positive attitude towards it.

This provides a good illustration of the importance of the normative component of the theory of planned behaviour. Smoking provides another. Smokers have, in the past, been influenced to give up through education about its potential health consequences or because of the development of actual health problems. However, smokers are currently in the minority and many are now giving up, not for health reasons, but because of the growing climate of public disapproval and increasing imposition of smoking restrictions. It is worth noting that legislation only usually takes place once the majority of public opinion is in favour of a particular course of action. The law which made the wearing of seat-belts compulsory was successfully introduced once public opinion supported it, and this increased compliance from about 60 per cent to over 90 per cent virtually overnight.

Normative pressure may be exerted in a number of ways, which include verbal expressions (telling people what we think) and a variety of non-verbal behaviours which signal our attitudes (approval or disapproval) towards the behaviour of other people.

Exercise

You invite friends round for dinner and one of them appears to be drinking too much. How might you signal your disapproval to her and to the other guests without actually saying aloud what you are thinking? Do you think that the guest in question will notice? If not, why not?

Not only are our attitudes culturally shaped through socialization processes, such as child-rearing, schooling and professional training, but most of us are socialized from an early age to respond quickly to public expressions of approval and disapproval. Insensitivity to social expectations and social cues can lead to behaviour which is interpreted by others as antisocial. Antisocial behaviour can lead to social isolation and depression. This is why social skills training is an important component in the management of those with learning disabilities and mental health problems.

Minority groups within society can form subcultures which have their own set of social norms. Members of such groups may be resistant to mainstream public opinion. A good example is that of teenage girls, among whom smoking is increasing. Health promotion for this group needs to include the creation of anti-smoking media images which have direct appeal to them. Sadly, smoking advertising is currently rather better at promoting a positive image of smoking than health promotion is at promoting a negative one.

Cognitive dissonance

A persuasive explanation for congruence between the three components of attitudes (affective, cognitive and behavioural) was offered by Leon Festinger (see Gross 1992: 532–5) in his theory of **cognitive dissonance**. Cognitive dissonance is a state of tension which occurs when an individual holds two or more cognitions that are psychologically inconsistent. For example, the belief that 'heavy drinking causes liver damage' may be inconsistent with the knowledge that 'I drink heavily'. A range of options is available to the individual to reduce or eliminate this state of dissonance, which includes:

1 Give up drinking altogether.
2 Reduce the dissonance by cutting down or changing to a low-alcohol brand.
3 Justify the behaviour by providing reasons why I am not susceptible to drink-related illness (for example, my grandfather drank like a fish and lived happily until he was 92).
4 Underestimate how much I actually drink.
5 Pretend (to others and myself) that I don't care.
6 Blame others for my drinking.
7 Gain support from mixing with other drinkers.

The last five responses are maladaptive because they are likely to lead to potentially harmful outcomes and some of these may be seen as irrational. In Freudian terms, some responses could be described as ego-defensive, since they employ defence mechanisms such as rationalization or denial. It may be difficult to persuade people to change their behaviour if they use these types of argument or defences to justify continuing with unhealthy lifestyles.

Persuasion

Theories of attitude change tend to centre around issues related to persuasion. Politicians, health educators and marketing firms all use techniques of persuasion in an attempt to influence attitudes on the assumption that this will affect the way that people behave. Health professionals use individual or group communication aimed at persuading individuals to change, while health promoters also use the mass media for purposes of mass persuasion. In fact, health promotion is based upon techniques of persuasion (see Downie et al. 1990).

There are six basic steps in the persuasion process:

1 The target must see or hear the message – the sender usually selects the medium (television channel, radio network, newspaper, magazine, leaflet, etc.) to ensure this happens.
2 The target must pay attention to the message – attention is selective, so the message must be attention-catching.

3 The target must understand the message – this may depend upon their level of knowledge and education, compared to the complexity of the message.
4 The target must accept the message's conclusion – this is less likely if it conflicts with long-standing beliefs or messages from other sources.
5 The target must remember the new knowledge and retain the new attitude – this is more likely to happen if significant others share similar attitudes, or if the issue is maintained in the public domain.
6 The target must translate their new attitude or behavioural intention into action which they must then sustain – this is probably the most difficult bit (see the smoking cessation programme outlined in Chapter 4).

Exercise

Daily kite-flying is being promoted as the latest way to a long and healthy life. The evidence is persuasive and you agree that it would be good for you. List the reasons which might induce you to give it a try. List the reasons which might stop you from trying it at all. You decide·to give it a go. Consider all the factors which might eventually influence you (a) to continue this hobby or (b) to give it up. How many of these factors are related to the original persuasive argument about health? How many of these relate to social factors and influences?

The sender of the message

There are certain features of message senders which have been identified as likely to influence their persuasive power:

- Are they credible? Is there evidence that they are expert on the issue? In general, health professionals can establish their credibility and trustworthiness through their professional position and qualifications.
- Are they trustworthy? Do they have anything to gain by persuading others?
- Are they attractive? Does the sender appeal to you?

Doctors may be perceived by some patients to have more credibility in relation to issues concerned with health than other health professionals, even when this is not actually justified (for example, on issues relating to diet or type of exercise).

It is often argued that health professionals should act as role models in terms of healthy lifestyles. However, there is evidence from social psychology to suggest that messages are more persuasive if the sender argues from a position which is apparently opposed to their self-interest. It could therefore be argued that a heavy drinker will take more notice of advice to cut down from a former alcoholic or heavy drinker rather than a teetotaller.

The attractiveness of the communicator is more influential for relatively trivial messages, than for serious ones. Nevertheless, health promoters may wish to pay attention to the smartness of their personal appearance to signal their professionalism and trustworthiness and to signal the positive value of a healthy image. It may be useful to use well-known personalities for mass media appeals, so that the public will pay attention to them and identify with them.

Exercise

Imagine you are in hospital recovering from an accidental back injury. You know that you are substantially overweight and have previously tried to lose weight unsuccessfully, but do not associate your weight with your accident. You are advised to go on a weight-reducing diet as part of your recovery programme. Does it make any difference *who* tells you this? For example, a wiry physiotherapist? An occupational therapist with a back problem? An overweight nurse? An attractive radiographer? A doctor whom you know smokes? Any of them? Consider how you might respond to each. How are you likely to feel and what action are you likely to take when you get home? Compare your responses to those of someone who is heavier or lighter than you are.

The nature of the message

The first issue to consider in relation to the message is whether it should appeal to logic or to the emotions. There is still a vigorous debate about whether or not fear appeals are effective. Using the health belief model, it would appear that fear appeals work by raising the individual perceptions of personal vulnerability.

Drink-driving campaigns, for example, frequently use shock tactics and appear to have some success. However, it is not clear if this is because potential drinkers see the adverts and decide not to drink and drive, or because significant others see the adverts and exert pressure on them not to drink or not to drive. Also, the early HIV/AIDS campaigns used fear tactics – remember the coffin? However, it is unlikely that this had much effect, since it was not directed at personal vulnerability. Although members of the homosexual community certainly did modify their behaviour, this probably occurred after friends of theirs had become ill or died.

There are suggestions that high fear appeals can result in the engagement of defence mechanisms or avoidance, rather than behaviour change. Alternatively, people may absorb high fear messages and worry about them, but not actually do anything about them. In order to take effective action, individuals must know what to do and how to do it. Messages must therefore be accompanied by clearly specified advice about effective actions.

Rational arguments appear to be more effective when the issue is important and unfamiliar to the audience, whereas if the importance of an issue is perceived to be low, or its familiarity high, emotional appeals may be more persuasive. In fact, human beings have a strong tendency to focus upon salient individual situations or incidents which have strong emotional appeal, rather than statistical or epidemiological evidence which has strong rational appeal. This is why a more recent campaign against HIV/AIDS featured individuals with whom different target groups would identify (for example, Peter is white, heterosexual and has never taken drugs). Television is the best medium for making emotional appeals, since emotional images are stronger when they combine sight, sound and movement. On the other hand, the printed media are probably better for presenting rational arguments. Rational arguments appeal intellectually to those with a higher level of general education and it may be important to target these categories in the early stages of a new campaign through broadsheet newspapers and professional journals.

A related issue concerns the presentation of one-sided versus two-sided arguments. A well-informed audience is more likely to be persuaded by two-sided arguments because they will be aware of the counter-arguments and will wish to see these addressed. A less well-informed audience is likely to be confused by two-sided arguments and it may be better to present them with a single point of view.

There are frequently situations in health care where individuals are asked to make quick decisions on the basis of complex considerations. Take the example of the expectant mother who is asked if she wishes to have a screening test for congenital abnormalities in her unborn child. If she has the test, what are the options if it is positive? If she chooses not to have the test, what are the potential consequences for her and her family? It is not the role of the health professional in this situation to influence her decision. However, the way in which the issues are presented may prove to be persuasive. Some relevant points are considered below.

Order of presentation

The importance of primacy and recency effects has already been discussed in Chapter 5. It is possible for health professionals unwittingly to influence a client's decisions by the order in which the issues are presented. Aronson (1988) pointed out that, in the United States, the judicial system may actually prejudice the case for the defence because the prosecution presents their case first and sums up last, thus gaining benefit from both primacy and recency effects.

Discrepancy between the argument and audience opinion

The greater the discrepancy between the argument being presented and the individual's current attitudes, the less the degree of attitude change is likely to be. Aronson (1988) suggested that alternatives for those confronted with discrepant messages are:

1 They can change their opinion.
2 They can induce the communicator to change his or her opinion.

3 They can seek support for their original opinion from supporters.
4 They can convince themselves that the communicator is untrustworthy or uncreditworthy.

Exercise

Think of something you really enjoy doing. Imagine that 'an expert' comes up with research to suggest that this may have long-term harmful effects. How do you feel about this? What is your initial response? What are you likely to do about it in the short term?

Complexity and presentation of the message

A simple piece of research was undertaken by Chaiken and Eagly (1976) in which students participated in legal debate. The case was presented to them in plain English or 'legalese', either verbally (in a speech) or as text. The students' understanding of the case under each condition was subsequently evaluated. It emerged that simple messages were easily understood in any format. Difficult messages were difficult to follow when presented as a speech, but not in a printed format. The reason for this is probably that individuals are able to read and comprehend the message at their own pace. As a result of this, students who heard the difficult message where not persuaded by the argument presented. Quite clearly, limited comprehension leads to limited persuasion.

The moral of this message for health care appears to be that, where complex information is given to patients, it should be provided in written (or possibly taped) format so that they can take it away and study it at their leisure.

Censorship, bias or selection

Cultural attitudes and expectations pervade all aspects of our lives through the media, reference groups, peers, parents, education and training. As a result, we are all 'primed' to be receptive to certain messages and to resist others. This may help to explain why it is difficult for health professionals to persuade lay individuals, particularly those from different ethnic or social groups, to adopt behaviours which do not conform to their own deeply held beliefs.

Censorship and bias are an integral part of any society or culture. Our use of language helps to ensure this. For example, middle-class bias may be determined from an individual's accent. The current emphasis on 'political correctness' may be an attempt to reduce labelling and prejudice (see below), but it may be regarded by some as a form of censorship. One person's 'commonsense' attitude may be seen by others as bigotry. It is helpful to understand the beliefs of those with whom we hope to communicate and to use these as the starting point for health education.

This will help to reduce accusations of bias and enhance the likelihood that persuasive messages will be attended to and taken seriously.

Audience/target effects

Selective attention

In a small study by Kleinhesselink and Edwards (1975), university students completed a questionnaire concerning their attitudes to the legalization of cannabis. They then listened to a broadcast, through headphones, that contained seven strong (irrefutable) arguments and seven weak (refutable) arguments in favour of legalization. Constant static noise made listening difficult, but the students could press a button to reduce this. Those who favoured legalization pushed the button significantly more often when strong arguments were presented; those who opposed legalization pushed the button significantly more often when weak (refutable) arguments were presented. The conclusion of this study was that individuals pay more attention to messages which support their own beliefs. This, of course, is entirely in keeping with cognitive dissonance theory.

Social comparison theory (Festinger 1957) proposed that individuals deliberately seek validation of their own attitudes and beliefs by attending to those who hold ideas similar to their own, and distancing themselves from those who hold different beliefs or attitudes. Thus some social groups may be difficult to penetrate by those who are seen as outsiders. Health educators need to find novel ways of gaining acceptance for health messages by such groups. For example, one way of getting health messages across to teenagers is by 'peer tutoring', whereby older pupils, particularly those who are high on 'street cred', are trained to teach younger pupils about important health issues such as drug misuse or safe sex.

Self-esteem and education

People with low self-esteem do not place high value on their own ideas and are therefore more likely to be compliant (though they are more likely in the long term to comply with members of their peer group than with health professionals). People with high self-esteem are more likely to question and challenge, but may be persuaded by rational argument. It has already been indicated in Chapter 6 that high self-esteem is linked to perceptions of self-efficacy and internal locus of control, such that people who feel in control of their own lives are more likely to feel good about themselves. Education is an important source of self-efficacy because it provides people with essential knowledge and life skills. Basic education is therefore an essential prerequisite for health education.

In the current debate about population control, it has been argued that women who have little education and little control over their lives have little incentive to limit the size of their families. Those who are better educated and who have opportunities to improve their situation through their own contribution have an incentive to limit time spent in child-bearing. Persuading women to use contraception is of little use if the pressure to produce more children in order to contribute to the family income is greater than their need to limit the number of children in order to save demands on a limited family budget; nor is it of use if women are powerless against male attitudes which value fertility as evidence of masculinity. Empowerment means more than sending persuasive messages and free condoms. It is probably no coincidence that countries with the lowest birth rates have the highest rates of educated female wage earners. General education is an important prerequisite for health education, while economic incentives cannot be ignored.

Immediacy of action and endurance of the message

The longer the time gap between persuasion and action, the more likely it is that other factors will intervene, and the greater the chance that the target will find counter-arguments. The message quickly loses its effect. Therefore, people need to be persuaded to take immediate action. The evangelist movement has capitalized on this by inviting members of the audience to make an immediate commitment. Another example is the salesman who requires an immediate signature. It has now been recognized that instant decisions may be regretted and the law provides a cooling off period to prevent this type of hard sell. However, psychologists sometimes use contracts to confirm their clients' commitment to an agreed behaviour change.

Once prompted, the new attitude must be sustained in order to preserve the behaviour change. Therefore, health promotion is more likely to be effective if a message or media image is maintained in the public domain over a long period of time. Mass campaigns are largely ineffectual unless the impetus is maintained (see Taylor 1991). Individuals will need to find sustained rewards from their new lifestyle if they are to find it as attractive as their old one. This is more likely to arise from new activities, social relationships or habits than from feeling healthier. Unfortunately, feeling good, like any other pleasure, is soon taken for granted.

Who complies?

Eiser and Gentle (1989) conducted a postal survey in which they asked people to identify their participation in a range of health-related behaviours, together with their attitudes towards health publicity. They used statistical grouping techniques which identified three types of attitude towards health campaigns, including 'irrelevance' and 'responsibility'. They found that those who smoked tended to score higher than non-smokers on 'irrelevance', indicating that smokers appear to reject health messages because they are perceived not to have any personal relevance for them. They also scored low on 'responsibility', indicating that they believe it is their right to do as they wish, and not society's right to tell them what to do. However, not all of Eiser and Gentle's results were in the expected direction. For example, people who jogged actually scored lower on 'responsibility' than non-joggers indicating that, like smokers, they believe that health is their own business. Nevertheless, those who took more exercise tended to see health campaigns as more relevant. Overall, those who engaged in healthy activities (those who did not smoke or drink heavily, took more exercise and ate healthy foods) were more likely to identify health campaigns as relevant than those who were engaged in unhealthy activities, which is worrying for health promoters.

Exercise

What motivates people to take up healthy exercise? What motivates people to persevere with exercise once they have started? How much does this have to do with health promotion? Get together with colleagues and brainstorm the main costs and benefits of taking regular exercise. What factors contribute to the variety of opinion?

Ley (1988) presented research findings which suggest that compliance is often poor among health professionals. For example, hospital-acquired infections cost the NHS a large amount of money each year. The main way in which infections are spread is from the hands of health professionals. Yet several researchers have found that compliance with desirable hand-washing practices among nurses is poor. Slade *et al.* (1990) found that the frequency of hand-washing improved only slightly, even though knowledge of its importance was assessed to be extremely good, following a vigorous hospital campaign. Why do you think this is? Can you think of any other ways that compliance with hand-washing might be improved?

 ## Obedience

Persuasion is a process of reasoning which is deliberately designed to promote compliant behaviour. However, there are other social processes which influence this type of behaviour. The psychologist Stanley Milgram was interested in how Hitler was able to induce mass obedience to engage in extreme acts of cruelty during the Second World War. He set up a famous experiment which had far-reaching implications. Milgram (1963, in Gross 1994: ch. 6) advertised for volunteers to take part in an educational experiment at Harvard University. On arrival, each volunteer was introduced to another participant (in fact a stooge) and lots were ostensibly drawn to identify who would be the 'pupil' and who would be the 'teacher'. In fact, the volunteer always took the part of the teacher. The teacher was told by Milgram to press a button, which would give the pupil an electric shock as a punishment if he made a mistake. The shocks were seen to increase in intensity from 15 to 450 volts, the upper range being clearly marked 'danger'. It came as a shock to Milgram, and to the public, that

26 of the 40 teachers continued, with encouragement, to give shocks of up to 450 volts even though the pupils had progressed through protests and screams and by this time were quiet. No subject terminated the experiment below 300 volts. (Note that in Britain the standard household voltage is 240 V.)

The following factors have subsequently been shown to influence obedience in this type of situation:

- The legitimacy or status of the authority figure – when conducted at a less well-known institution, obedience was less, although still alarming.
- The proximity of the victim – obedience was less likely when the victim was in the same room, rather than behind a glass screen.
- The proximity of the authority figure – obedience was less likely when the experimenter was in another room and gave instructions by telephone.
- Personal characteristics of the target – some people appear to be more defiant and less conformist than others.
- Habit – some people respond automatically to authority cues.
- Social rules of commitment – having agreed to participate in the experiment, the volunteers felt obliged to do as they were asked.

In case health care professionals are wondering what this has to do with them, a subsequent 'real-life' experiment was conducted by Hofling *et al.* (1966; see Gross 1992: 582). A drug marked 'Astroten 5 mg; maximum dose 10 mg' was placed in the drugs cabinet on a ward. An experimenter purporting to be a psychiatrist telephoned the ward and asked the nurse in charge to give a named patient 20 mg of this bogus drug. An observer intercepted the nurse before she reached the patient; 21 of 22 nurses complied with the instruction even though there was no written prescription, the drug exceeded the safe dose (11 claimed not to have noticed this), and neither the drug nor the 'doctor' had previously been heard of by the nurse. Could this type of problem occur today?

Exercise

Imagine that you are working on a unit where a patient is attending for an investigation which requires the routine administration of a relatively harmless drug. The Trust rules state that you are not allowed to give any drug without a doctor's written prescription. A new doctor has forgotten to write it up for one patient. He tells you over the telephone to go ahead and administer it to the patient and he will sign up later. What do you do? What are the possible implications of your course of action?

In 1994, three teenagers from a local school were spending their first day in an accident department as part of a work experience programme when they were told by a doctor, who assumed they were nurses, to stitch up a patient's wound. They did!

The strength of this type of social influence is evident in everyday life. There are few of us who have not fallen for the sales patter of the authoritative salesman. Parents, teachers, bosses, generals and dictators all appeal to obedience, frequently without the need to use force. One of the main reasons for introducing diploma or degree level training for all health care professionals is to raise awareness about these effects, to encourage questioning and not to accept answers uncritically. Challenging authority does not make individuals popular, which is one of the main reasons why there are so few dissenters!

Conformity

The tendency to conform with members of our own social group provides another important source of social influence. The creation of fashions by the marketing industry is an illustration of the importance of **conformity**. In fact, any mother who has tried to buy her youngster a pair of cheap trainers which does not bear the appropriate prestige brand name will testify to this.

Conformity has been demonstrated in a number of classic psychology experiments. One conducted by Solomon Asch in the early 1950s (see Gross 1992: 563–8) involved male college students who were told that they were participants in an experiment about visual judgement. They were asked to match the length of the line shown on a card with one of the three shown on a separate card (as shown in Fig. 9.2). This appears to be an extremely straightforward and unambiguous task. However, when the student was unknowingly placed in a room with confederates of the experimenter who selected the wrong line, one-third of students gave the same 'wrong' answer which had been given by the confederates; 70 per cent of students conformed on at least one occasion. Only a minority remained independent in the face of this type of group pressure.

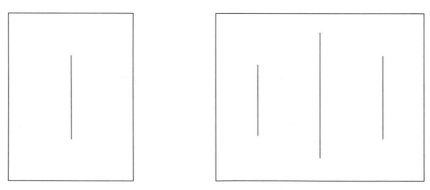

Figure 9.2 Presentation similar to that used in the Asch experiment on conformity. Participants were asked to match the length of the line on the left-hand card with one of the lines on the right-hand card.

Exercise

Imagine you are a student nurse working on a first clinical placement. You are asked to take a routine blood pressure. You are not confident and are unable to detect meaningful sounds at the first attempt. What are you likely to do? You try again, and this time are reasonably confident with the result. However, it is much lower than this patient's previous recordings. What do you do? The pressure is checked by another nurse who, having first checked the chart, confidently announces a pressure in line with previous recordings. You try again and obtain another low recording. How do you feel? What do you do?

The above situation is one which every nurse will have encountered at some time. It serves to highlight the potential lack of objectivity in even something as simple as a blood pressure recording. If we are really honest, few people take a blood pressure without first checking the previous recordings – what are the implications of this?

A number of important factors have been shown to be influential in determining the likelihood that an individual will conform:

1 Conformity to the views and behaviour of other people is more likely when the information available upon which to make a decision is ambiguous or sparse. This is true of many situations in health care.
2 The desire for social approval (normative influence) can, in many cases, override other aspects of judgement.
3 We are more likely to conform with the views of others if we perceive their expertise to be greater than ours. Novices may be correct, but it is the views of experts which are generally heeded.
4 Conformity is more likely in those with low self-confidence, poor self-esteem and poor perceptions of self-efficacy. Conformity is less likely where confidence, self-esteem and perceived self-efficacy are high.
5 Non-conformity and non-compliance are also higher among those with a strong desire for self-expression. This is often regarded by others as attention-seeking behaviour, evidence of eccentricity, or simply 'being difficult'. In other words, being different rarely attracts social approval. Nevertheless, non-conformity can lead to new and creative ways of thinking about problems and some of our most famous scientists and best-loved public figures actually fit into this category (usually in retrospect).

It has been suggested that the failure of individuals to act on their own beliefs because they believe that others know best or are in control of the situation, is an important causal factor in a number of major disasters, including Chernobyl, where the local maintenance team appear to have assumed that a team of experts from Moscow knew what they were doing and were in control of the situation, even though they could see that the dials clearly registered danger levels (Reason 1987).

Exercise

You have just fallen in love for the first time, but you know that your partner has had a number of previous short-term relationships. You have used a condom until now, but your partner now tries to persuade you that this is no longer necessary. Your head tells you that there is a risk of catching a sexually transmitted disease, but your heart wants to believe your partner. What are you likely to do? What are the factors which are likely to influence your decision in this context? Does it make a difference if you are male or female and, if so, why? You insist on using a condom, but your partner seems less keen and your friends tell you that there is no risk because your partner is such a nice person. What do you do next time you meet your partner?

Bystander apathy

Conformity is one of the factors which has been blamed for what has been termed bystander apathy. This was highlighted in the USA when a young woman, Kitty Genovese, was brutally murdered outside a block of flats. Her cries for help during a half-hour period were heard by a large number of people, yet no-one telephoned for the police. Latané and Darley (1968) subsequently staged a series of emergencies to examine the circumstances in which bystanders are likely to intervene, and those where they fail to intervene (see Gross 1992).

Exercise

You are travelling alone using the underground and find yourself in a carriage with 10 other people. A middle-aged man with a ruddy complexion and rather grubby appearance enters the carriage and then gradually collapses to the floor. Nobody else takes any action. Some bury their heads in their newspapers. What do you do? Suppose that the man was smartly dressed and had a pale complexion. What would you do? Why might his appearance make a difference?

The following factors appear to be influential in determining action (Latané and Darley 1970):

- People are more likely to act if there are cues to the seriousness of the situation from other people. Thus once one person initiates action, others will follow.

- The larger the number of strangers present who do nothing, the less likely an individual is to intervene. In this situation, each individual assumes that someone else will take the necessary action.
- People fail to act if they perceive themselves incapable of doing anything to help. Conversely, they are more likely to act if they feel they can do something useful to help.
- People are less likely to act in ambiguous situations. For example, people in British society are likely to ignore someone lying on the pavement because the individual might be drunk, rather than ill.
- People are more likely to take action if they have the opportunity to discuss the situation with other people first.

Helping actions are also influenced by the perceived 'deservedness' or culpability of the victim. This may relate to a 'just world' hypothesis in which people are presumed to get what they deserve. Modern-day dilemmas centre upon the homeless who beg on our streets and the extent to which they are perceived to be the victims or the scroungers of our society. These dilemmas frequently relate to moral issues within a society or culture. Helping behaviour is often influenced by the belief that the action would result in social approval. The desire for social approval leads some people to publicize their helping activities, while others shun publicity.

The extent to which the 'victim' is perceived to be attractive is likely to influence helping behaviour. People are more likely to give to charities which portray appealing images than those which elicit distaste or disgust. Perhaps this is why animal charities do so well. Major charities, such as Mencap and Scope (formerly the Spastics Society), have changed their images to promote a more attractive impression of those they support, in the hopes of generating more positive attitudes and appealing to more potential donors.

Social desirability is an important consideration for anyone undertaking research involving people, whether this involves experiments, questionnaire surveys, observation or in-depth interviews. Individuals invariably try to interpret what is required of them and may modify their responses as part of their own impression-management. This is why social researchers frequently use false cover stories. The need to obtain informed consent poses a dilemma for health care researchers who need to balance ethical considerations on the one hand against the need to reduce social desirability bias on the other.

Non-verbal behaviour

It has been suggested that an important way in which affective and behavioural components of attitudes are communicated is through **non-verbal communication**. We often 'give away' our feelings or attitudes without being consciously aware of doing it and this is referred to as 'leakage'.

Studies of patient satisfaction with health care have repeatedly shown that interpersonal aspects of care are central to patients' perceptions of quality of care. It is not just what we do, as health professionals, it is the way that we do it. The *Patients' Charter* has recognized the need for personalized care, and the introduction of primary nursing, as opposed to task-oriented nursing, is one way of helping to ensure that hospital in-patients receive this. In fact, there is evidence to suggest that primary nursing increases nurses' job satisfaction as well as patient satisfaction. Positive and negative attitudes such as satisfaction or dissatisfaction, pleasure or anger, approval or disgust, are likely to be revealed through non-verbal signals. Negative attitudes can be hard to disguise.

Exercise

Imagine that you meet someone you like very much. Write down how an independent observer (out of earshot) would recognize what your feelings are. Now imagine you meet someone that you dislike very much. Write down how the observer might recognize your dislike.

We reveal a lot about ourselves through non-verbal communication. For example, we signal confidence or nervousness through our body posture, hand movements, facial expression, tone of voice and speed of delivery. Likewise, we can use these cues to recognize confidence or stress in patients.

Exercise

List all of the ways in which you might recognize anxiety in a patient. How do non-verbal signals of anxiety vary from one individual to another?

Role management

Once we are aware of these non-verbal signals, we can modify them to create an outward impression which may be quite different from our inner feelings. Ervine Goffman (1971) described a 'dramaturgical theory' which regards social interaction as akin to a theatrical performance. The issue of self was discussed in some detail in Chapter 3, but has equal relevance to social psychology. Goffman actually used the example of the doctor to illustrate his dramaturgical model, although similar processes occur in all professions or jobs. As a medical student, learning to become a doctor involves more than just acquiring medical knowledge and skills. It requires looking and behaving like a doctor, developing a bedside manner and instilling confidence into patients. The image of the doctor is maintained by the patients who have traditionally tended to hold doctors in awe, and by the nurses who prepare the patients, the trolleys, carry out commands and have adopted an inferior role. Anyone who has witnessed the traditional consultant's 'round' will be left in no doubt about the doctor's role and the doctor–nurse relationship, although attitudes have recently begun to change.

People often try to enhance their own self-image by making selective social comparisons between their own performance and those who are less skilful. Some people actually try to manipulate others into an inferior role; for example, by ridiculing them in front of others or ignoring their suggestions, which Goffman called 'altercasting'.

Goffman outlined how we use props to sustain our role through **impression management**. Clothes, hairstyle, make-up, perfume and briefcase are all examples of the props we use to portray the public image we wish to present. The doctor's stethoscope and white coat are part of the props used to create the image of the doctor. In fact, the performance of some 'bogus' doctors has been so convincing that it has taken a long time before their lack of medical knowledge or expertise has exposed them.

Each profession has its own set of props and behaviour into which newcomers are initiated and socialized. These are learned more by modelling than through formal instruction, although it is hoped that once we understand how these processes occur, we can recognize these aspects of our own behaviour and seek to modify these deliberately where necessary. In fact, role development is a process of learning how to look and how to behave, testing and readjusting the role. Each health professional develops a distinctive role which involves certain norms and expectations of social behaviour.

> **Exercise**
>
> Describe the role which characterizes your own profession. What are the behaviours and props associated with it? What makes your own profession similar to, or distinctive from, other health care professionals?

The ease with which individuals adopt the roles expected of them, and some potentially dreadful consequences which can follow, were illustrated by Zimbardo and his colleagues in the Stanford University prison experiment (Haney *et al.* 1973, in Gross 1994: ch. 7). The basement of a university building was converted into a prison with three cells, a solitary confinement cell and an observation room for prison guards. Twenty-one volunteers were screened prior to participation to ensure their physical and mental stability. Nine were **randomly** assigned to the role of prisoner. The remainder were appointed as guards and were given uniforms, mirror sunglasses, a wooden baton each and a whistle. The experiment had to be terminated after 6 days because the guards had become increasingly aggressive and sadistic, while the prisoners became passive and negative. Toileting had become a privilege, rather than a right. Upon their release, the prisoners expressed relief. However, the guards had enjoyed the power and found it difficult to relinquish this.

Similarities with the situation described above are to be found in a variety of institutional settings. Another of Goffman's famous works, *Asylums* (Goffman 1968a), reported on a study of staff and inmate behaviour in a variety of institutions. His observations are disturbing, but are of relevance to any institution or service in which one group of 'professionals' has power or control over another group of people such as patients.

Exercise

There have been periodic examples in the media during the 1980s and 1990s where attention has been drawn to neglect or cruelty which has taken place in institutions for the most vulnerable in society: children, the mentally ill, those with learning disabilities and the elderly. Look up at least one of these. Try to explain why this might have happened. What steps might be taken to prevent such atrocities?

The famous study by Rosenhan in the early 1970s 'On being sane in insane places' (Rosenhan 1973, in Gross 1994: ch. 18) clearly illustrates how a diagnosis of mental illness can be difficult to shake off once established. This type of scenario will be familiar to those who have seen the film 'One Flew Over the Cuckoo's Nest', in which a reporter who claimed to 'hear voices' was admitted to a mental institution with a diagnosis of schizophrenia. Although he reported no further symptoms, his behaviour, including note-taking, was all interpreted as further evidence of his insanity. Once a diagnosis is established and a label placed on the patient's condition or state, it can become very difficult to change and this is true of physical as well as mental health care.

Exercise

It has been reported in the media that the incidence of psychotic illnesses (those which involve abnormal thoughts and behaviour) are more common among those belonging to ethnic minority groups in Britain. Debate the possible reasons for these findings.

Stereotyping, stigma and prejudice

Stereotyping is a process of attaching certain attributes to an individual according to group membership. Sociologists generally refer to this as labelling. It draws upon certain salient characteristics which have some foundation in fact or experience. However, these characteristics are often exaggerated and are generalized at the expense of individual character-istics. Stereotypes may be based upon national or regional charac-teristics, race, gender or age-related characteristics, or may be related to common features such as height, weight or hair colour. For example, people with red hair have fiery tempers and Scots people are mean. Some of these stereotypes are positive, but many are negative.

Stereotyping is a convenient form of shorthand or schema for describing people. However, negative stereotypes can lead to group polarization and prejudice. The stereotype can become a self-fulfilling prophecy. A famous classroom experiment conducted by Rosenthal and Jacobson (1968) illu-strated this. Pupils were given an intelligence test and a randomly selected group of them were subsequently identified to their teachers as 'spurters'. When the intelligence tests were repeated at the end of several months, these children were found to have made significant improvements over the rest of the children. The best explanation of this is that the teachers responded differently to them, giving them more encouragement and positive feedback. This research was instrumental in questioning the con-ventional wisdom of school selection at the age of 11, and the practice of streaming.

Expectations are extremely powerful sources of unconscious bias in human behaviour. They have already been referred to in relation to the placebo effect (see Chapter 8). They can have a confounding influence on a range of 'pure' scientific research, simply because the researcher almost always approaches the study with certain hopes or expectations. When Rosenthal (1966) randomly classified laboratory rats as 'bright' or 'dull' before giving them to students to train to run in a maze, he found that those classified as bright far outperformed those classified as dull. This was probably because the students behaved quite differently in the way they handled and encouraged the 'bright' rats. When the subjects of research are human, as in social research, the possibilities of expectation effects are that much greater. This is one reason why data obtained in the social sciences contains much more variability than the physical sciences, and why different researchers rarely obtain identical results, even when they follow the same written protocol, and why identical treatments given by different people often vary in their effect.

Prejudice and attribution theory

The negative effects of stereotyping can be demonstrated in all aspects of life. Negative stereotypes lead to prejudice: the combination of negative beliefs, attitudes and discriminatory behaviour towards those in a particular target group. Prejudice is associated with 'isms', such as racism, ageism, sexism and class divisions.

Prejudice may be understood in terms of attribution theory. The prin-ciples of attribution theory have been covered in Chapter 4, although its significance is best understood within a social context. Prejudice involves the tendency to make negative global and stable dispositional attributions about negative characteristics such as poverty or ill-health, rather than attributing these to environmental or situational causes. This inevitably leads to 'victim-blaming'. Thus the poor are blamed for their poverty and the sick for their illness.

> **Exercise**
>
> A pleasant middle-aged man is admitted with severe circulatory problems which may require below-knee amputation. How do you feel towards him? You then find out that he is still a heavy smoker, even though his doctor has repeatedly told him about the consequences of not giving up. Now how do you feel towards him? You later find that he has experienced substantial personal and financial problems which he blames for his inability to give up. Does this influence your attitude towards him?

When things go well in our own lives, we tend to attribute our success to our own actions; however, when things go badly, we tend to blame external environmental or situational factors, or other people. When we make judgements about other people's lives, we tend to reverse this. The general tendency to overestimate dispositional or personal (internal) factors and underestimate the influence of environmental or situational factors *in other people* is termed the **fundamental attribution error**. The fundamental attribution error is probably one of (if not the most) important concept within psychology, because it represents such a common mistake which can have far-reaching consequences.

Blaming the unemployed for being lazy at a time when there are over three million people looking for jobs is an example of this. Blaming poverty on fecklessness when surveys indicate that low benefit levels and wages are the main factor is another example. Looking for personality traits to account for anxiety, instead of situational factors, may (or may not) be another.

Goffman (1968b) referred to negative labels based upon personal characteristics as **stigma**. This has been discussed in some detail in Chapter 3. Once a stigmatizing label such as 'neurotic' or 'depressive' has been attached to an individual, it is difficult to remove it. The term **psychosomatic** innocently means an illness which involves both physical and psychological contributory factors. However, it is frequently misinterpreted and used as a label for a physical disorder which has no detectable medical cause and which, by default, is considered to have a psychological origin. The correct term for this is actually **psychogenic**. Asthma was included in this category before the importance of allergens and pollutants as causal agents was identified. It is worth remembering that once a stigmatizing label has been recorded in a patient's medical records, it stays there, right or wrong, often without the patient's knowledge, and can influence subsequent care.

Case study: Susan

Susan was a former nurse and the mother of a 3-year-old boy (her second child) whose physical and mental development was seriously delayed. Susan was anxious to find out what was causing her son's problems and to obtain the best help for him. She felt that the local paediatrician had been less than helpful and asked him for another specialist's opinion. When this was not forthcoming, Susan requested help from her doctor and health visitor. She could not understand why, for months, she kept coming up against negative attitudes. On looking through the child's notes, the health visitor found a letter from the paediatrician containing the words, 'this mother is manipulating the social services', which was curious because the family was not even known to the social services at that time.

In the field of health care, there is increasing emphasis on self-care, personal responsibility for health and the need for empowerment. One of the less fortunate consequences of this becomes apparent when the individual becomes ill or fails to get better. It is all too easy to suggest that it is the fault of the individual for failing to take advice or action and not to look at the social environment in which that individual lives, which restricts opportunities for taking personal action and effectively disempowers him or her. For example, the failure of a mother to provide adequate nutrition for her children when living in bed-and-breakfast accommodation; or the failure of a young teenager to insist that her older and more assertive male partner should use a condom.

Exercise

An elderly gentleman is diagnosed as diabetic and advised to change his diet in line with current advice (no sugar, increased fibre, fresh fruit and vegetables, low saturated fat). Subsequent blood tests indicate that he is not adhering to his diet. Consider the dispositional, environmental and situational factors which may be influencing his behaviour. How might knowledge of these factors enable you to help him to make the necessary adjustments? (You may wish to refer back to some of the issues raised in Chapters 4 and 6.)

The importance of individualized and holistic care

One of the main antidotes to prejudice and victim-blaming in health care is an emphasis upon individualized, client-centred care, which recognizes individual beliefs, expectations and needs during the assessment, planning and implementation of care strategies. Another is the use of a holistic assessment which takes into account the environmental and situational constraints and resources within which the individual patient is functioning.

The medical model of care has fostered the creation of stereotypes by fitting individuals into diagnostic categories. This can lead to **depersonalization** in which the individual patient is regarded as 'the leg in bed 22', rather than Mrs Griffiths, aged 66, who has a fractured femur, lost her husband and only daughter in an accident 6 years ago, has recently moved to a second-floor flat with no lift and has left her much loved cat in the care of a new neighbour. The medical model has tended to emphasize dispositional factors in accounting for responses to sickness or trauma. Thus Mrs Griffiths' fussing and anxiety may be attributed to her personality, rather than genuine worry about her cat and how she will cope on her own when she goes home.

Geriatric medicine has long carried a stigma of its own, along with the tendency to depersonalize older people. The rewards of elderly care become apparent once an individualized approach to care is adopted. Task-oriented care focuses mainly upon the rituals of toileting, bathing, changing and feeding. Individualized care of the elderly can elicit rich rewards in revealing anecdotes and personal history. Reminiscence and life review appear to raise self-esteem and self-confidence and stimulates motivation to participate in self-care. The tasks become less onerous for the patient and the nurse as they engage in a closer rapport. Some tasks may become less necessary as the nurse and patient work together to identify reasons for particular behaviour patterns.

The remainder of this chapter includes a brief introduction to the contribution of social psychology to the issues of effective leadership, group processes and the management of change, with particular reference to health care.

Leadership

Just as the rise of Hitler and the aftermath of Hitler's Germany stimulated Stanley Milgram's work on obedience, so it stimulated Kurt Lewin to study the issue of leadership. In fact Lewin had escaped from Nazi Germany before the war and initiated a series of studies with colleagues in America. One of the first such studies was the effect of authoritarian, democratic and *laissez-faire* leadership. You might note the similarities between these terms and those used later to describe parenting styles (see Chapter 4 on the development of locus of control). Parents are, after all, leaders and some of Lewin's early work involved children (see Pennington 1986). The evidence seems to suggest that democratic leadership encourages participation, engenders a sense of ownership and commitment within the group and generally leads to higher morale, friendliness, cooperation and productivity (see also Broome 1990). Authoritarian leadership is based upon coercion and is generally associated with lower morale among the group or workforce. It can be useful in order to achieve an important task quickly, but may place undue stress upon some members of the group. Most people prefer to work under strong but democratic leadership. Although psychological research has focused upon personality characteristics of good leaders, leadership is substantially a matter of skill and involves techniques which do not necessarily come naturally. Hence the importance of good management training for all those who undertake a management or leadership role within the NHS, particularly at a time of rapid change.

Group interaction

A useful way of making decisions can be to set up a committee or working party to debate the issues and reach a conclusion. However, this can be a hazardous process. Kogan and Wallach (1967; see Pennington 1986) described a group phenomenon which they termed 'risky-shift'. They found that groups were frequently likely to take riskier decisions than individual members of the same group. One of the possible reasons for this was the dispersal of responsibility for the outcome of the decision. However, these and other researchers noted a shift towards caution under certain circumstances and this led Moscovici and Zavalloni (1969) to propose a theory of 'group polarization'. The hypothesis of this theory is that the average group decision will tend to be more extreme, but in the same direction as the average of the individual responses before the group came together.

Irving Janis, a psychologist who was also famous for his work on stress, was prompted by a major international incident to investigate these group decisions in more depth. The incident was the American decision, in 1961, to support the unsuccessful invasion of Cuba in what became known as 'The Bay of Pigs' disaster. This prompted the Cuban missile crisis of 1962 and led the president, Kennedy, to admit that a dreadful mistake had been made by his highly expert group of advisers. But how and why? Janis (1982) analysed the group processes involved and proposed that they had been victims of **groupthink**. Some of the main symptoms of groupthink are identified below:

1 Illusion of invulnerability – positions of power can lead people to believe that they cannot be proved wrong.
2 Collective rationalization – unrealistic assessments are supported by 'rational' arguments, sufficient to convince other group members.
3 Belief in the inherent morality of the group – the belief that they are in the right and good must triumph.
4 Stereotypes of out-groups – outsiders are often automatically classified as 'bad guys' or enemies who must therefore be in the wrong.
5 Direct pressure on dissenters – dissenters are silenced and this discourages critical evaluation. Certain group members may take the initiative to reduce dissent (by persuasion or coercion) and foster an illusion of unanimity. Silence is interpreted as support.

Butler et al. (1994) described the British Government decision in 1991 to introduce the 'poll tax' as an example of groupthink at its worst. Local authority treasurers, opposition members and Nigel Lawson (all out-group members) predicted that it would be tremendously expensive, if not impossible, to collect and warned of huge losses in revenue. However, government officials and ministers under Mrs Thatcher (the in-group) were single-minded in their determination. The result was an enormous cost to the taxpayer and a system which had to be replaced within 2 years. You may care to consider examples of NHS expenditure which might fall into this category.

Work on group composition suggests that small groups which include a mixture of individuals with different skills and viewpoints are probably more effective in reaching an informed decision. Heterogeneous groups are less likely to succumb to groupthink. Group size is another important consideration. It is rare for groups exceeding twelve members to be effective, whereas a group of five or six people facilitates the active participation of each member. The chairperson needs to play an important and impartial role in encouraging each member to voice their opinions, and encourage the debate of any doubts.

The potentially divisive nature of social groupings, in terms of intergroup discrimination and prejudice, was demonstrated by Tajfel (1970, in Gross 1994: ch. 11). Tajfel's work suggests that members of a group generally work towards maximizing profits or rewards for members of their own group (the in-group), often at the expense of other groups (out-groups). An illustration of this is to be found in the vigorous defence of pay differentials within industry, or the battle between specialities for scarce resources within the NHS. Within the NHS, examples of in-group/out-group conflict have been found in the relationships between enrolled nurses and registered nurses, hospital and community, private and NHS, or between units in different localities. At a time when interdisciplinary cooperation is increasingly necessary, professional identity can form a barrier to the delivery of quality patient care. The 'multidisciplinary team' may need to become the in-group of the future.

Organizational management and change

The NHS has, for the last 25 years, been undergoing intensive periods of rapid change. Most recently, the introduction of a market framework has led to some major shifts in the philosophy of care delivery. Staff at all levels have been involved in this and it has in many instances caused stress (see Chapter 6) and poor morale. Effective leadership and management of change has never been a more important issue than it is in today's NHS.

A detailed discussion of change management is outside the scope of this book, and the reader is directed towards Broome (1990) and Teasdale (1992) for a more detailed appraisal of the issues. The most successful change management strategy is one in which staff are encouraged to participate in goal setting and decision making as members of a multidisciplinary team, and to take personal responsibility for their own workload, while at the same time receiving the support and resources necessary to achieve the agreed goals. This gives all individuals a sense of control and confidence and contributes towards a good atmosphere. This affects inter-personal care and is an important determinant of patient satisfaction. These aspects of ward environment have been identified as an important influence on patient behaviour in mental health settings (Moos 1974).

The traditional organizational structure within the NHS, as with many other large organizations, has been a hierarchical one in which the important decisions are made at the top and instructions filter down, if they are lucky, to those at the bottom. In this type of situation, those who actually provide patient care may feel that they have little opportunity for involvement in (or influence on) decision making, limited autonomy and little control. An advantage of a flat (as opposed to a pyramidal) manage-ment structure is that communications and involvement at all levels are easier. The problem is that career progression may be seen to be limited.

Exercise

Construct a chart of the organizational structure of the unit in which you are currently working. Locate where decisions about care management policies are made and indicate the direction in which these decisions are transmitted. Identify your own feelings about working in this environment and the morale of those who work with you. How do you think these relate to the extent of personal control and support available?

Authoritarian leadership can tend to promote a ritualistic task-oriented approach to patient care where the main aim is to get the job done. The most effective manager is generally one who is prepared to delegate responsibilities, encourages individual expertise and ownership of innova-tions, and facilitates interdisciplinary collaboration, while at the same time ensuring that staff are adequately supported in taking the risks which are inevitably involved in changing practice. Staff frequently blame low morale on personality clashes or high workload, when the underlying reason is the leadership style of managers, the structure and philosophy of the organization and inadequate resources (Webb 1989). These issues are closely related to the issues of stress and coping in organizations which were referred to in Chapter 6 and the reader is encouraged to refer back to these for further reading.

Summary

- Theories of attitude and attitude change, including cognitive dissonance theory, are outlined.

- Theories of persuasion, including factors relating to the sender, the message, the medium and the receiver, are outlined and considered in relation to health promotion.

- Research into obedience, compliance and bystander apathy are presented and their relevance to health care and health professionals highlighted.

- The significance of non-verbal communication is considered, with particular reference to role development and impression management among health professionals and patients.

- The importance of roles in determining attitudes and behaviour is highlighted.

- Stereotyping, prejudice and their significance in health care situations are emphasized, with particular reference to the fundamental attribution error, depersonalization and the importance of individualized and holistic care.

- Research into issues of leadership and group processes are presented, with particular reference to organizational structure and change within health care.

Further reading

Argyle, M. (1983) *The Psychology of Interpersonal Behaviour*, 4th edn. Harmondsworth: Penguin.

Atkinson, R.L., Atkinson, R.C., Smith, E.E. and Bem, D.J. (1993) *Introduction to Psychology*, 11th edn. Orlando, FL: Harcourt Brace Jovanovich. Chapter 18.

Goffman, E. (1968) *Asylums – Essays on the Social Situation of Mental Patients and Other Inmates*. Harmondsworth: Penguin.

Gross, R.D. (1992) *Psychology: The Science of Mind and Behaviour*, 2nd edn. London: Hodder and Stoughton.

Gross, R.D. (1994) *Key Studies in Psychology*, 2nd edn. London: Hodder and Stoughton.

Taylor, S.E. (1991) *Health Psychology*, 2nd edn. New York: McGraw-Hill. Chapter 10.

EPILOGUE

This book has set out to introduce the reader to a variety of psychological theories and research which are relevant to health care. These final comments highlight some of the issues which you may have become aware of during the course of reading about the different approaches which have been described. They also identify some additional areas of relevance for future developments in health care. By now you will have sufficient knowledge to think critically for yourself about the issues which are raised.

You may have observed that applied researchers interested in particular aspects of the human condition, such as facial disfigurement or pain, or those within psychology who have developed theories in relation to development or social interaction, have often been influenced by a particular model of psychology. This should not prevent you, as a consumer of psychological theory, from examining the potential implications of adopting one approach, rather than another. The fact that an important theorist or group of researchers has used a particular model does not imply that this is the only applicable model, nor that it is necessarily the best one. There are criticisms of all of the models which have been presented and some of these are considered below.

Humanistic psychology, while intuitively appealing, makes no claim to be scientific and offers few hypotheses which have been tested experimentally. Therefore, if you like humanistic propositions you will accept them, and if you don't, you'll reject them. The danger of this is that practice is often supported by subjective opinion, rather than objective 'fact'. You might wish to question how it is that a school of psychology which was founded by individuals who were primarily interested in the treatment of those with psychological problems, has been used to form the basis of models (such as nursing models) for the treatment of people whose primary problem is a physical or a social one. As you will see from the comments below about other models, these observations do not imply that humanistic psychology is any less valid than the other schools of theory within psychology. Indeed, the humanistic framework, with its emphasis on the needs of the individual, appears to lie at the heart of dealing with many of the problems related to attachment, persuasion, stereotyping, prejudice, stigma, leadership and organizational stress, which were identified within developmental and social psychology and stress research.

Psychoanalytic theory is, to a great extent, untestable. Indeed, the theory itself could be used to suggest that rejection of it by individuals or groups is, in fact, a defence mechanism against a method which may well unleash disturbing emotions. Psychoanalysis emerged from an interest in physical problems which were thought to have psychogenic origins. Therefore, although they are 'person-centred', one might question the wisdom of applying theories which were derived from 'abnormal' situations to normal human psychology. Nevertheless, both the humanistic and psychoanalytic models attempt to deal with the complexity of human feelings and this has intuitive appeal to all of those who work in the caring services. Both models emphasize the importance of the relationship between the therapist and patient and the importance of good interpersonal skills, much of which is supported by objective research from developmental and social psychology, and stress theory and research.

Behaviourism emanated from experiments in the animal behaviour laboratory and the theories of learning which it has generated have been heavily criticized for their lack of relevance to complex human thought processes, and behaviour in complex situations. Recent research has led to cognitive reinterpretations of behavioural learning and it is difficult to distinguish between contemporary behavioural and cognitive psychology. Behaviour modification was successfully applied in the 1960s and 1970s within institutions for the mentally ill and mentally handicapped. One of the reasons why it has subsequently gained a poor reputation may be because of the inappropriate use of 'time out' as a punishment (although this was attributable to bad practice, rather than to poor psychological theory). There were also doubts that changing behaviour, alone, improved quality of life for the individuals concerned. Nevertheless, learning principles from behaviourism are still very influential in understanding human behaviour and influencing changes in individual behaviour. Most contemporary approaches to behaviour change which incorporate behaviourist principles are now termed 'cognitive–behavioural' (for example, see the smoking prevention programme of David Marks outlined at the end of Chapter 4). This is because these approaches recognize the ability of most individuals to use behaviourist principles to analyse and change their own behaviour in whatever situation they happen to be in. In fact, most cognitive–behavioural therapies are based upon humanistic principles of client-centred care in which clients are encouraged to identify their own goals. The main difference is that therapy retains a sense of direction and purpose which is negotiated and agreed between the client and the therapist throughout their period of contact (or contract).

Much of cognitive psychology is actually open to criticisms which are similar to some of those levelled at behaviourist, psychoanalytic and humanistic psychology. Much of the early research into human memory, for example, was based upon the presentation of very simple stimuli. Subsequent research has confirmed the relevance of some of the theories which were derived from this early work, but many of the theories which have been produced to account for perception and memory for complex material are not open to confirmation or refutation through research. Future work in psychophysiology and computer science may, or may not, offer support for much of this work. On the other hand, cognitive therapies (those which are based purely upon the deliberate manipulation of thought processes) have emerged from therapy with emotionally disturbed patients and there is little evidence that these are any better or any worse than therapies which are located within other models of psychology.

As far as therapeutic approaches to dealing with psychological distress and psychological problems are concerned, these are usually based upon the preferences of the individual therapist. Sometimes the therapist chooses to include aspects of different approaches to suit the needs of individual clients, using an eclectic approach. Those who use psychology to inform their practice are likely to select the approach which is most appealing to them. However, it is likely that individual clients will also seek out the approach which most suits their own particular coping style. Some people naturally prefer the structured problem-solving approach afforded by the cognitive–behavioural approach, while others prefer the self-reflective approaches offered by humanist or psychoanalytic approaches. It is important that clients with psychological problems should be involved in choosing the approach which best suits them, rather than having to conform to the whim of the person allocated to care for them. The act of negotiating what the individual wants, in any health care situation, is central to good patient care. In fact, the evidence, such as it is, suggests that what makes a 'good therapist' is not so much the type of approach they use but their interpersonal skills.

It is hoped that in reading this book you will now be aware that many psychological problems are not something which can only be dealt with by a psychologist or specialist therapist. Much of the anxiety, depression and maladaptive coping that we encounter as health professionals is not the actual problem but the consequence of common everyday problems experienced by ordinary people (see Mirowsky and Ross 1989). These include physical illness, personal relationship problems and losses, and problems of social inequality such as those related to education, employment, housing and access to health care. We do not have to be psychologists to listen to clients' problems and support them in addressing these issues. The very act of providing an empathetic ear is likely to help to reduce distress and suffering in the immediate situation. However, we do need to recognize the boundaries of our abilities to help people and know when to seek expert help or advice. It is likely that working within a multidisciplinary team of people who each have a different perspective on a particular patient problem will produce better and more effective solutions for patients. This is why an informed knowledge of psychology and its potential applications, together with research-based evidence, is essential for all health care professionals.

The future success of health care within the NHS is likely to depend upon working together within multidisciplinary teams which will jointly assess patient needs and manage patient care in hospitals and, increasingly, the community. The disease model, with its emphasis upon treatment and compliance, is already giving way to a health empowerment model, in which the focus is upon personal control, self-care and the maintenance of social roles and functions. The context of the patient will eventually cease to be the hospital bed and will increasingly focus upon the home, the family, the local community and the workplace. You should now be able to justify the importance of this shift in emphasis using psychological theories and research. You should also be aware of the difficulties which are likely to confront the health educators and promoters of the future.

Central to the application of psychological principles in practice (regardless of the model used) are the skills of listening, empathizing, negotiating with and advising individuals. In other words, interpersonal skills. Interpersonal skills are the vehicle by which psychology is applied in practice, whatever the context. The majority of patient complaints about health care can be traced back to poor interpersonal skills on the part of health care professionals. The manner in which care is provided is usually the only way that lay people have to judge the quality of the service provided. This is why social and interpersonal skills are likely to be the core multidisciplinary subject for all medical and health care professionals in the future.

Therapists working in the professions allied to medicine, and nurses and midwives working in the community, have traditionally had greater opportunities to provide individualized care than nurses and midwives working in hospital wards and departments. This is changing. The implementation of primary nursing and government directives towards the introduction of the named nurse and named midwife have provided the impetus for a more individualized approach to care. A recent innovation in health care, designed to improve practice and care, is the setting up of 'development units', many of which have been supported and funded by the King's Fund. Although they may be termed a 'nursing' or 'midwifery' development unit (NDU or MDU), they usually support a multidisciplinary approach to care. Their main aim is to 'develop' research-based practice. You will, by now, be well aware of the theory and research which justifies and supports the need for client-centred, as opposed to task-oriented, care. As you will see from this book, support for an individualized approach to care can be found in all models of psychology. Research suggests that it is beneficial for staff and patients, providing adequate support is available within the organization in which they work. We hope that this book will help all of those working in the caring professions to understand that they have personal needs which should be met within their area of employment if they are to provide sustained and effective care.

Our main hope in writing this book has been to stimulate the same level of interest and excitement which psychology has brought to us, as nurses. We have each come to this book with preferences for different psychological models. It will be interesting to see if you can detect, from your reading, who has written which chapters by examining the biases in approach. However, we hope that you will now see that all aspects of psychology have something relevant to say about all aspects of practice in health care. We hope that better use of psychology will be made in future as medical staff combine with nurses, midwives and therapists to appreciate its potential contribution to the provision of quality health care for all.

GLOSSARY

Active versus passive coping: doing something versus doing nothing when faced with a potentially threatening situation.

Actual self: term used in humanistic and social psychology, and incorporated in the repertory grid, to describe the self as one believes oneself to be and the attributes one believes one has. Usually reflects reality, but occasionally distorted (as in anorexia), in which case it may be associated with psychological problems.

Adaptation: the process of change in beliefs and behaviour which results from experience.

Amnesia: memory loss; may be retrograde (an inability to remember past events that were previously recalled) or anterograde (an inability to recall anything which has occurred after a traumatic event or stage in a disease process).

Anxiety: a state of emotional tension which exists within an individual when perceived internal and external demands are not matched by the perceived ability to meet those demands.

Approach/avoidance: refers to ways of coping with threatening situations, either by confronting the situation or by avoiding it.

Attachment: from developmental psychology with psychoanalytic influence (Bowlby); theory that the development of a close relationship (attachment) between mother and child is necessary for the psychological well-being and adjustment of the developing individual. Later extended to include types or qualities of attachment and attachment relationships throughout the lifespan.

Avoidance: behaviour which avoids contact with undesirable or feared stimuli or consequences. Maladaptive if it disrupts lifestyle or leads to dependence on others.

Behaviourism: a behaviourist approach to psychology which is based upon operant conditioning principles.

Behaviourist: a school of psychology in which principles of learning are derived from observing changes in behaviour in response to certain stimuli or conditions.

Bereavement: a perception of loss by death.

Biopsychosocial: combination of biological, psychological and social systems (as opposed to considering each system separately).

Bipolar: refers to a scale of measurement which has both a negative and a positive pole (e.g. semantic differential scale, Likert scale).

Bonding: from developmental psychology; refers to a theory that a close attachment between mother and baby soon after birth is important in the development of the future relationship between mother and child.

Burnout: a chronic state of stress in health and social care workers which negatively affects their ability to be able to care for other people.

Catharsis: a term from psychoanalysis which is used to describe the therapeutic release of emotions.

Causal attributions: from social psychology; the beliefs that individuals have about the causes of events, whether due to internal factors (self) or external factors (powerful others, or luck, fate or chance).

Classical conditioning: from behaviourist psychology; simple associative learning by which a previously neutral stimulus, such as a sound, sight, smell or sensation, stimulates a reflex behavioural or emotional response.

Cognition: thought processes; includes perception, memory and information processing.

Cognitive appraisal: term from stress/coping theory (Lazarus 1966); used to describe the thought processes by which an individual determines the degree of threat associated with an event and what to do about it (how to cope with it).

Cognitive dissonance: from social psychology (Festinger 1957), but appears to have psychoanalytic influences; refers to a state of tension which exists when an individual holds two or more conflicting beliefs. The theory proposes that the individual will take any of a variety of possible actions in order to reduce this tension.

Cognitive therapy: cognitive treatment for psychological disorders, such as anxiety and depression, in which individuals are encouraged to change the way they think about events.

Compliance: from social psychology; term used to describe actions which are in accordance with the instructions of or wishes of others.

Conditioned emotional response: from behaviourist psychology (classical conditioning theory); a negative emotional response (such as fear) which is usually triggered by a noxious or threatening stimulus but which, through association, becomes triggered by a neutral (non-threatening) stimulus.

Conditioning: from behaviourist psychology; a simple form of associative (or conditional) learning which takes place (usually at an unconscious level) in response to external events or stimuli.

Conformity: from social psychology; the natural propensity of individuals to act in accordance with the behaviour or beliefs of others.

Constructs: from humanistic psychology (Kelly 1955); bipolar belief systems, the means by which people construe (interpret and understand) the world.

Coping: from Lazarus' (1966) theory of stress; cognitive and behavioural responses to situations which are based upon an appraisal of threat or potential harm.

Coping strategies: term used in cognitive theories of stress to describe the cognitive and behavioural actions which are used by individuals to reduce actual or potential sources of perceived threat. May be conscious (rational) or unconscious (reflex or habitual).

Coping style: term used in theories of stress to describe the relatively stable ways in which an individual normally deals with situations and events.

Cue: from behaviourist psychology; a stimulus event, situation or context which acts as a trigger for a certain response.

Daily hassles: term used in stress research to describe minor events which disrupt or interrupt daily life or routine and impose demands upon coping resources.

Decentre: from developmental psychology (Piaget); the ability to see things from the point of view of another person.

Defence mechanisms: from psychoanalysis (Freud); term used to describe a range of unconscious processes, such as denial, which defend the ego from unmanageable threat and emotions (such as anxiety).

Delayed gratification: from social learning theory; refers to the delay (or wait) between the promise of a reward and its receipt. Some individuals are better able to tolerate delay, while others require immediate gratification for their needs.

Denial: from psychoanalysis (Freud); a defence mechanism in which an individual who is faced with a problem claims that nothing is wrong.

Depersonalization: from social psychology and sociology (Goffman 1968a); the treatment of an individual as an object, rather than a person. Sometimes a symptom of burnout among health care professionals.

Depression: cognitive–behavioural definition (according to the theory of learned helplessness; Seligman 1975); a psychological state involving cognitive, motivational and emotional deficits.

Drive-reduction: a behaviourist theory of motivation (Hull 1943) which proposes that behaviour is motivated by the reduction of inner states of tension (e.g.

eating is driven by hunger). Similar to Freud's pleasure principle and Maslow's need theory.

Eclectic: term used to describe a form of psychological therapy which draws from a variety of different psychological models.

Egocentrism: from developmental psychology; seeing things only from a personal point of view (the inability to see things from the point of view of others).

Emotion-focused coping: term used in stress theory (Lazarus and Folkman 1984), but derived from psychoanalysis; a method of coping which is designed to contain or reduce unpleasant emotions, such as anxiety. Includes defence mechanisms.

Empiricist: follower of a traditional school of psychology rooted in the belief that all knowledge is derived from experience.

Episodic memory: memory for past events or situations, usually based upon visual images.

Fight or flight response: from psychophysiology (Cannon 1932); behavioural response to threat noted in animals and used to describe the immediate physiological response to stress in humans.

Functional analysis: from behaviourism; a systematic analysis of the immediate causes and consequences of problem behaviours (including anxiety), usually by the use of a diary. Enables the therapist and client to plan changes to modify behaviour and reduce the occurrence of the problem.

Fundamental attribution error: from social psychology; wrongly blaming individuals for their problems, rather than the situation they are in. Occurs very frequently in health and social care.

Generalization: from behaviourism; term used to describe the process by which a behaviour which occurs in response to one stimulus (event or situation) subsequently occurs in response to other similar stimuli.

Grief: the emotional response to feelings of loss.

Groupthink: from social psychology (Janis 1982); describes a type of group interaction which can sometimes lead an expert group to make spectacularly wrong decisions.

Habitual (habit): a behaviour which takes place regularly and no longer requires conscious (deliberate) consideration (behavioural psychologists refer to this as overlearning).

Health locus of control: from health psychology (Wallston *et al.* 1978); locus of control beliefs with particular reference to responsibility for maintaining health and dealing with illness.

Health psychology: a new applied discipline within psychology which is concerned with theory and research relating to beliefs and behaviour in health and illness.

Hierarchy of needs: from humanistic psychology (Maslow 1970); a model of identifiable human needs in which lower-order (basic) needs must be satisfied before higher-order needs can be met.

Homeostasis: an adaptable state of balance within the body's physiological systems, disrupted by disease and external stressors.

Iatrogenesis: from medicine; unintentional consequences of medical treatment, medically induced side-effects which include maladaptive behaviours.

Ideal self: from humanistic psychology; the self that an individual would like to be and the attributes or qualities they would like to have.

Impression management: from social psychology; the deliberate use of language, body language, make-up, clothing or other 'props' to influence the attitudes and behaviour of others towards us.

Imprinting: a rapid type of learning that occurs in some animals very soon after birth.

Information: term used by Gibson (1966), in relation to his theory of direct perception, to describe relatively stable or changing structures which are manifest in internal and external stimuli or events and picked up by the senses. The means by which we can identify what things are and what is happening to us and around us.

IQ (intelligence quotient): a standardized measure of cognitive ability based on the ratio of mental age to chronological age, with a population average score of 100.

Law of effect: a rule which states that if a response occurs in the presence of a particular stimulus which is rewarded, this will result in the response being more likely to occur when the stimulus is next encountered.

Learned helplessness: from behaviourist psychology (Seligman 1975) and later adapted using attribution theory; uncontrollability – a combination of cognitive, motivational and emotional deficits, resulting from experience, which leads individuals to believe that their actions have no control over outcomes. Used as a model for human depression (among others).

Life events: term used in stress research to describe events in the lives of individuals which require adjustment or change.

Likert scale: a measure of attitude commonly used in psychological research, based upon a measure of agreement versus disagreement.

Locus of control: from Rotter (1966) and combining behaviourist principles with socio-cognitive (attribution) theory; relatively stable causal attributions (beliefs) that outcomes are dependent either on personal actions (internal LOC) or external forces such as powerful others or luck, fate or chance (external LOC). Later divided into three orthogonal (unrelated) dimensions: internal, powerful others and chance (Levenson 1974).

Loss: unpleasant or painful sensations associated with separation from a loved person, object, desired state or body part or function.

Maladaptation: from cognitive and behavioural theories of stress; responses to change which lead to adverse consequences for self or others (for example, they cause anxiety or depression, or impose unreasonable demands on members of the social network).

Mnemonic: term used to describe a technique of visual or verbal association to enhance retention in memory.

Modelling: from social learning theory (Bandura 1977); the learning of new patterns of behaviour by observing and mimicking others.

Mourning: the behavioural expression of grief, which is shaped by the cultural context.

Nativist: follower of a traditional school of psychology rooted in the belief that humans are born with certain unique abilities to organize knowledge and have special ways of responding to the environment.

Non-verbal communication: from social psychology; the conscious or unconscious use of body language, make-up, clothing or other 'props' to signal meaning or intention to other people.

Normative influence: from social psychology; refers to social influences on individuals to conform to what is accepted by the majority (the social norm) in terms of attitude, belief or behaviour.

Operant conditioning: from behaviourism; a simple form of learning in which voluntary responses are determined or shaped by immediate reinforcement or punishment, in a particular context. Sometimes termed instrumental conditioning.

Ordinal data: commonly refers to verbal rating scales of frequency or intensity, such as those used in attitude scales, in which numbers are assigned sequentially to the scale for the purposes of analysis, but the intervals between points on the scale cannot be assumed to be equal. For example, the interval between strongly agree (5) and agree (4) cannot be assumed to be the same as between agree (4) and neutral (3).

Overlearning: from behaviourist psychology; refers to the point in operant conditioning at which responses have become automatic or habitual.

Personal construct theory: according to Kelly 1955, a theory of personality in which people form hypotheses or constructs which determine the way they view the world.

Placebo: a dummy intervention (e.g. sugar pill or attention only) which induces a positive physiological effect (such as pain reduction).

Placebo effect: physiological response induced by expectation.

Preparedness: a nativist view within behaviourist psychology (Seligman 1971); refers to the innate propensity of a species to behave or respond in a particular way to certain stimuli (e.g. fear of snakes).

Primacy effect: term from memory research used to describe the phenomenon that information presented first tends to be remembered better than subsequent information.

Primary appraisal: term used in stress/coping theory (Lazarus 1966) to describe the cognitive process by which an individual determines if an event poses a potential psychological or physical threat. Followed by secondary appraisal to determine appropriate action.

Primary attachment figure: first significant lasting relationship formed by a baby with a care-giver, usually the mother.

Primary memory: term used to describe short-term or working memory.

Primary reinforcer: from behaviourist psychology and influenced by drive-reduction theory; a reinforcer which reduces a need directly (for example, food, which reduces hunger). *See also* secondary reinforcers.

Proactive interference: term from memory research; situation in which information received first interferes with memory for subsequent information.

Problem-focused coping: from cognitive psychology (Lazarus and Folkman 1984); responses to a threatening situation which are based upon a problem-solving analysis.

Procedural memory: memory for behaviour patterns, related to routine procedures and skills. Often retained when other forms of memory have failed (e.g. you never forget how to ride a bike).

Psychoanalysis: a method of investigation, theory of mind and method of treatment invented by Sigmund Freud.

Psychogenic: a disease or physical phenomenon which has a psychological origin. Mainly used in the context of psychoanalytic psychology. Sometimes incorrectly applied when there is no known medical cause for a physical symptom.

Psychoneuroimmunology: the study of the relations between psychosocial events and immunological parameters.

Psychosomatic: a term used to describe a disease or physical phenomenon (such as pain) which is caused by a combination, or interaction, of psychological and physical (somatic) factors.

Punisher: from behaviourism; a consequence which decreases the likelihood of a behaviour occurring again.

Punishment: from behaviourism; when used in operant conditioning, it refers to a consequence which decreases the likelihood of a behaviour occurring. Withdrawing attention is often a successful punishment, using this definition.

Randomized controlled trial (RCT): research method regarded as the gold standard for demonstrating the effectiveness of a medical or psychological intervention. Subjects are randomly allocated to an intervention group, or a control group which receives a placebo intervention. This controls for individual variations in response and the placebo or attention effect. Usually conducted blind so that the individual who administers the intervention or collects and analyses the data cannot introduce expectation bias.

Randomly: occurs by chance. Random allocation to sample groups in research eliminates systematic bias (e.g. ensures equal numbers of males and females, etc.). It may be achieved by drawing names out of a hat, but usually involves giving each potential subject a number and using random number tables to determine grouping.

Recency effect: term from memory research used to describe a situation in which information given last in a sequence is remembered better than previous information. *See also* the primacy effect.

Reference group: from social psychology; a group of people who share certain attributes and goals with an individual and with whom that individual closely identifies.

Reinforcement: from behaviourism; the provision of a consequence which increases the likelihood of a behaviour (note, this is not the same as rewarding, although rewards are often reinforcing).

Reinforcer: from behaviourism; a consequence which increases the likelihood of a behaviour (not necessarily the same as reward).

Repertory grid: from humanistic psychology; a method devised by Kelly (1955) for analysing the self concept, based upon personal constructs.

Representational theory: a theory of perception which proposes that visual stimuli are interpreted within the brain to form a mental representation of the external environment. This representation may be subject to interpretive bias.

Repression: from psychoanalysis; term used to describe a defence mechanism which involves the unconscious 'forgetting' of painful memories in order to protect the ego.

Retroactive interference: term from memory research used to describe a situation in which new information interferes with (alters or eliminates) memory for information previously received.

Rogerian counselling: from humanistic psychology (Carl Rogers); non-directive client-centred therapy for psychological problems in which the therapist provides an atmosphere of 'unconditional positive regard' to enable the individual to reflect on and solve their own problems and achieve personal growth.

Safety signal: from behaviourist psychology; an environmental cue which is associated with safety and security (as opposed to threat).

Schedule of reinforcement: from behaviourism; refers to the frequency or regularity with which reinforcement is offered or delivered.

Schema: from cognitive psychology (memory processes); a mental representation of an event or pattern of events which provides an understanding of what is happening.

Script: from cognitive and social psychology (memory processes); a mental representation of the sequence of behaviour which is usually followed in a particular situation (as though the individual was an actor in a play).

Secondary appraisal: from stress/coping theory (Lazarus 1966); the stage following primary appraisal in which the individual decides what resources are available to tackle a perceived threat and what action to take.

Secondary reinforcer: from behaviourism; a reinforcer which is associated with a primary reinforcer or can be used to obtain primary reinforcement (e.g. money).

Self: a concept which is central to humanistic psychology and used to refer to what constitutes 'I' or 'me'.

Self-actualization: from humanistic psychology; a process of attaining maximum personal growth.

Self-efficacy: from social learning theory (Bandura 1977); the belief that I could do something, and achieve a positive outcome, if I wanted to.

Self-esteem: a term used in humanistic psychology and social learning theory to describe feeling good about oneself.

Self-modification: developed from behaviourism and behaviour modification; the use, by individuals, of a system of rewarding themselves for certain behaviours in order to reinforce those behaviours (for example, treating oneself to a meal out as an incentive for completing an assignment).

Semantic differential scale: a useful bipolar psychological measure based upon the presentation of a series of positive versus negative words, for example:

happy I _ I _ I _ I _ I _ I _ I sad

Semantic memory: memory for words and language structures.

Sensitive period: from developmental psychology; a critical period of development during which certain environmental stimuli or experiences are likely to influence the course of future physical or psychological development.

Social cognition: from social psychology; thought processes which take place in, or are influenced by, the social context in individuals' lives and functions.

Social comparison theory: from social psychology, a theory which proposes that our self-identity is formed and maintained by comparing our own attributes and characteristics with those of others.

Social support: from cognitive, humanistic and social psychology; some aspect of the behaviour of other people which contributes to the psychological and physical well-being of an individual.

Stigma: from social psychology and sociology (Goffman 1968b); physical or behavioural attributes or distinguishing features which have a negative impact on the behaviour of others towards the afflicted individual.

Stimulus: used in behaviourist psychology to describe any external event which can be picked up by the senses (sight, sound, taste, smell, touch) and lead to a response.

Stimulus control: from behaviourist psychology; a situation where a behavioural response which is triggered automatically (unconsciously) by an environmental stimulus or cue (such as lighting up a cigarette with a cup of coffee).

Stressors: external events or conditions which pose an actual or potential physical or psychological threat to an individual.

Systematic desensitization: from behavioural psychology (Wolpe 1958); a systematic method of eliminating a conditioned emotional response in which the individual is gradually reintroduced to the feared object while maintaining full relaxation.

Threat: from stress theory; an environmental event or situation which is perceived to be potentially damaging to physical or psychological well-being.

Token economy: from behaviourism; a method of incentive, based upon secondary reinforcement, used in institutions or controlled environments to eliminate undesirable behaviours. Individuals are provided with tokens for exhibiting socially desirable behaviours, which they can then use to buy what they want. Originally used in mental institutions, but not dissimilar to the system of star rewards used with children in schools or the home.

Unconditional positive regard: from humanistic psychology and central to client-centred therapy; love and esteem which is freely given by one person to another and does not depend upon the way the other behaves.

Universal helplessness: associated with learned helplessness; the belief that neither I nor anyone else can do anything about my situation (hopelessness)

Vicarious reinforcement: from social learning theory; learning to expect personal reinforcement in certain situations by watching others being rewarded for similar actions in similar circumstances.

REFERENCES

Ainsworth, M.D.S., Blehar, M.C., Waters, E. and Wall, S. (1978) *Patterns of Attachment*. Hillsdale, NJ: Lawrence Erlbaum Associates.

Ajzen, I. (1988) *Attitudes, Personality and Behaviour*. Milton Keynes: Open University Press.

Ajzen, I. (1991) The theory of planned behavior. *Organizational Behavior and Human Decision Processes*, 50:179–211.

Ajzen, I. and Fishbein, M. (1980) *Understanding Attitudes and Predicting Behavior*. Englewood Cliffs, NJ: Prentice-Hall.

Alley, T.R. (1981) Head shape and the perception of cuteness. *Developmental Psychology*, 17:650–4.

Archer, J. and Winchester, G. (1994) Bereavement following death of a pet. *British Journal of Psychology*, 85:259–71.

Argyle, M. (1983) *The Psychology of Interpersonal Behaviour*, 4th edn. Harmondsworth: Penguin.

Aronson, E. (1988) *The Social Animal*, 5th edn. New York: W.H. Freeman.

Atkinson, R.L., Atkinson, R.C., Smith, E.E. and Bem, D.J. (1993) *Introduction to Psychology*, 11th edn. Orlando, FL: Harcourt Brace Jovanovich.

Ayllon, T. and Azrin, N.H. (1968) *The Token Economy: A Motivational System for Therapy Rehabilitation*. New York: Appleton Century Crofts.

Baider, L. and De-Nour, A.K. (1986) The meaning of a disease: An exploratory study of Moslem Arab women after a mastectomy. *Journal of Psychosocial Oncology*, 4(4):1–13.

Bailey, R. and Clarke, M. (1989) *Stress and Coping in Nursing*. London: Chapman and Hall.

Bandura, A.A. (1977) *Social Learning Theory*. Englewood Cliffs, NJ: Prentice-Hall.

Baumrind, D. (1967) Child care practices anteceding three patterns of preschool behaviour. *Genetic Psychology Monographs*, 75:43–8.

Becker, M.H. and Rosenstock, I.M. (1984) Compliance with medical advice, in A. Steptoe and A. Mathews (eds), *Health Care and Human Behaviour*. London: Academic Press.

Beecher, H.K. (1959) *Measurement of Subjective Responses*. New York: Oxford University Press.

Beisecker, A.E. (1988) Aging and the desire for information and input in medical decisions: Patient consumerism in medical encounters. *The Gerontologist*, 28(3):330–4.

Bem, D.J. (1967) Self-perception: An alternative interpretation of cognitive dissonance phenomena. *Psychological Review*, 74:183–200.

Benner, P. and Wrubel, J. (1989) *The Primacy of Caring: Stress and Coping in Health and Illness*. Menlo Park, CA: Addison-Wesley.

Berde, C.B. (1991) The treatment of pain in children, in M.R. Bond, J.E. Charlton and C.J. Woolf (eds), *Proceedings of the VIth World Congress on Pain*. Amsterdam: Elsevier.

Berk, L.E. (1991) *Child Development*, 2nd edn. Needhan Heights, MA: Allyn and Bacon.

Bernstein, D.A., Clarke-Stewart, A., Roy, E.J., Srull, T.K. and Wickens, C.D. (1994) *Psychology*, 3rd edn. Boston, MA: Houghton Mifflin.

Bibace, R. and Walsh, M.E. (1981) Children's conceptions of illness, in R. Bibace and M.E. Walsh (eds), *New Directions for Child Development: No. 14. Children's*

Conceptions of Health, Illness and Bodily Functions. San Francisco, CA: Jossey Bass.

Blackmore, S. (1989) A survey of general medical knowledge among university students: Its implications for informed consent and health education. *Senior Nurse*, 9(10):17–21.

Boore, J.R.P. (1978) *Prescription for Recovery*. London: Royal College of Nursing.

Bowlby, J. (1969) *Attachment and Loss: Vol. 1 Attachment*. London: Hogarth Press.

Bowlby, J. (1980) *Attachment and Loss: Vol. 3. Loss*. London: Hogarth Press.

Brewer, M.B. (1991) The social self: On being the same and different at the same time. *Personality and Social Psychology Bulletin*, 17:475–82.

Briner, R. (1994) Stress: The creation of a modern myth. Paper presented at the *Annual Conference of the British Psychological Society*, Brighton, March.

Broome, A. (1990) *Managing Change*. Basingstoke: Macmillan.

Brown, G.K. and Nicassio, P.M. (1987) Development of a questionnaire for the assessment of active and passive coping strategies in chronic pain patients. *Pain*, 31:53–64.

Bull, R. (1988) *The Social Psychology of Facial Disfigurement*. New York: Springer-Verlag.

Butler, D., Adonis, A. and Travers, A. (1994) *Failure in British Government: The Politics of the Poll Tax*. Oxford: Oxford University Press.

Callaghan, P. and Morrissey, J. (1993) Social support and health: A review. *Journal of Advanced Nursing*, 18:203–10.

Callaghan, D. and Williams, A. (1994) Living with diabetes: Issues for nursing practice. *Journal of Advanced Nursing*, 20:132–9.

Calnan, M. and Rutter, D.R. (1986) Do health beliefs predict health behaviour? An analysis of breast self-examination. *Social Science and Medicine*, 22:673–8.

Calnan, M. and Rutter, D.R. (1988) Do health beliefs predict health behaviour? A follow-up analysis of breast self-examination. *Social Science and Medicine*, 26:463–5.

Cannon, W.B. (1932) *The Wisdom of the Body*. New York: Norton.

Carroll, D. and Bowsher, D. (eds) (1993) *Pain: Management and Nursing Care*. Oxford: Butterworth-Heinemann.

Chaiken, S. and Eagly, A.H. (1976) Communication modality as a determinant of message persuasiveness and message comprehensibility. *Journal of Personality and Social Psychology*, 45:241–56.

Champion, V.L. (1984) Instrument development for health belief model constructs. *Advances in Nursing Science*, April, p. 81.

Cobb, S. (1976) Social support as a moderator of life stress. *Psychosomatic Medicine*, 38(5):300–14.

Cohen, F. and Lazarus, R.S. (1979) Coping with the stresses of illness, in G. Stone et al. (eds), *Health Psychology*. San Francisco, CA: Jossey Bass.

Cohen, M.Z., Tripp-Reimer, T., Smith, C., Sorofman, B. and Lively, S. (1994) Explanatory models of diabetes: Patient practitioner variation. *Social Science and Medicine*, 38(1):59–66.

Cohen, S. and Edwards, J.R. (1989) Personality characteristics as moderators of the relationship between stress and disorder, in R.W.J. Neufeld (ed.), *Advances in the Investigation of Psychological Stress*. Chichester: Wiley Interscience.

Cooper, C.L. and Payne, R. (eds) (1991) *Personality and Stress: Individual Differences in the Stress Process*. Chichester: John Wiley.

Cooper, C.L., Cooper, R.D. and Eaker, L.H. (1988) *Living with Stress*. Harmondsworth: Penguin.

Cox, T. (1978) *Stress*. London: Macmillan.

Curbow, B., Somerfield, M., Legro, M. and Sonnega, J. (1990) Self-concept and cancer in adults: Theoretical and methodological issues. *Social Science and Medicine*, 31(2):115–28.

Department of Health (1992a) *The Health of the Nation*. London: HMSO.

Department of Health (1992b) *The Patient's Charter*. London: HMSO.

Downie, R.S., Fyfe, C. and Tannahill, A. (1990) *Health Promotion: Models and Values*. Oxford: Oxford University Press.

Drettner, B. and Ahlbom, A. (1983) Quality of life and state of health for patients with cancer in the head and neck. *Archives of Otolaryngology*, 96:307–14.

Eiser, C. (1990) *Chronic Childhood Disease*. Cambridge: Cambridge University Press.

Eiser, C. (1993) *Growing Up with a Chronic Disease*. London: Jessica Kingsley.

Eiser, C. and Patterson, D. (1983) 'Slugs and snails and puppy-dog tails' – children's ideas about the inside of their bodies. *Child: Care, Health and Development*, 9:233–40.

Eiser, J.R. and Gentle, P. (1989) Health behaviour and attitudes to publicity campaigns for health promotion. *Psychology and Health*, 3:111–20.

Ellerton, M.L. and Merriam, C. (1994) Preparing children and families psychologically for day surgery: An evaluation. *Journal of Advanced Nursing*, 19:1057–62.

Engel, G.L. (1959) 'Psychogenic' pain and pain-prone patient. *American Journal of Medicine*, 26:899–918.

Erikson, E.H. (1963) *Childhood and Society*, 2nd edn. New York: Norton.

Evans, A. (1994) Anticipatory grief: A theoretical challenge. *Palliative Medicine*, 8:159–65.

Facione, N.C. (1993) Delay versus help seeking for breast cancer symptoms: A critical review of the literature on patient and provider delay. *Social Science and Medicine*, 36(12):1521–34.

Fallowfield, L. with Clark, A. (1991) *Breast Cancer*. London: Routledge.

Fallowfield, L. and Hogbin, B. (1989) Helping patients with cancer – the provision of audiotapes of the 'bad news' consultation. Paper presented at the *International Conference on Health Psychology*, Cardiff, September.

Festinger, L. (1954) A theory of social comparison processes. *Human Relations*, 7:117–40.

Festinger, L. (1957) *A Theory of Cognitive Dissonance*. Stanford, CA: Stanford University Press.

Fleissig, A. (1993) Are women given enough information by staff during labour and delivery? *Midwifery*, 9:70–5.

Flor, H., Kerns, R.D. and Turk, D.C. (1987) The role of spouse reinforcement, perceived pain and activity levels of chronic pain patients. *Journal of Psychosomatic Research*, 31(1):251–9.

Fordyce, W.E. (1976) *Behavioural Methods for Chronic Pain and Illness*. St. Louis, MO: C.V. Mosby.

Friedman, M. and Rosenman, R.H. (1974) *Type A Behavior and Your Heart*. New York: Knopf.

Furnham, A. (1994) Explaining health and illness: Lay perceptions on current and future health, the causes of illness, and the nature of recovery. *Social Science and Medicine*, 39(5):715–25.

Gibson, J.J. (1966) *The Senses Considered as Perceptual Systems*. Boston. MA: Houghton Mifflin.

Gillmore, M.R. and Hill, C.T. (1981) Reactions to patients who complain of pain: Effects of ambiguous diagnosis. *Journal of Applied Social Psychology*, 11(1):13–22.

Goffman, E. (1968a) *Asylums – Essays on the Social Situation of Mental Patients and Other Inmates*. Harmondsworth: Penguin.

Goffman, E. (1968b) *Stigma – Notes on the Management of Spoiled Identity*. Harmondsworth: Penguin.

Goffman, E. (1971) *The Presentation of Self in Everyday Life*. Harmondsworth: Penguin.

Goren, G.C., Sarty, M. and Wu, P.Y.K. (1975) Visual following and pattern discrimination of face-like stimuli by newborn infants. *Pediatrics*, 56:544–9.

Graham, H. (1993) *Smoking Among Working Class Mothers*. Report, Department of Applied Social Studies, University of Warwick.

Gregory, R.L. (1970) *The Intelligent Eye*. London: Weidenfeld and Nicholson.

Gross, R.D. (1992) *Psychology: The Science of Mind and Behaviour*, 2nd edn. London: Hodder and Stoughton.

Gross, R.D. (1994) *Key Studies in Psychology*, 2nd edn. London: Hodder and Stoughton.

Hack, T.F., Degner, L.F. and Dyck, D.G. (1994) Relationship between preferences for decisional control and illness information among women with breast cancer: A quantitative and qualitative analysis. *Social Science and Medicine*, 39(2):279–89.

Haight, B.K. (1988) The therapeutic role of a structured life review process in home-bound elderly subjects. *Journal of Gerontology: Psychological Sciences*, 43(2):40–4.

Hallett, R. (1991) Psychological preparation for surgery: A critical analysis. *Clinical Psychology Forum*, February, pp. 20–4.

Harkapaa, K., Jarvikoski, A., Mellin, G., Hurri, H. and Luoma, J. (1991) Health locus of control beliefs and psychological distress as predictors for treatment outcome in low back pain patients: Results of a 3-month follow-up of a controlled intervention study. *Pain*, 46:35–41.

Hayes, N. (1994) *Foundations of Psychology*. London: Routledge.

Hayward, J.C. (1975) *Information – A Prescription Against Pain*. London: Royal College of Nursing.

Helman, C.G. (1978) 'Feed a cold, starve a fever': Folk models of infection in an English suburban community, and their relation to medical treatment. *Culture, Medicine and Psychiatry*, 2:107–37.

Heurtin-Roberts, S. (1993) 'High-pertension': The uses of a chronic folk illness for personal adaptation. *Social Science and Medicine*, 37(3):285–94.

Hobfoll, S.E. (1988) *The Ecology of Stress*. New York: Hemisphere.

Hodges, J. and Tizard, B. (1989) Social and family relationships of ex-institutional adolescents. *Journal of Child Psychology and Psychiatry*, 30:77–99.

Hofling, K.C., Brotzman, E., Dalrymple, S., Graves, N. and Pierce, C.M. (1966) An experimental study in the nurse–physician relationship. *Human Development*, 13:90–126.

Hollway, W. (1984) Gender differences and the production of subjectivity, in J. Henriques, W. Hollway, C. Urwin, C. Venn and V. Walkerdine, *Changing the Subject: Psychology, Social Regulation and Subjectivity*. London: Methuen.

Holmes, T.H. and Rahe, R.H. (1967) The Social Readjustment Scale. *Journal of Psychosomatic Research*, 11:213–18.

Holzman, A.D. and Turk, D.C. (1986) *Pain Management: A Handbook of Psychological Treatment Approaches*. New York: Pergamon Press.

Hull, C.L. (1943) *Principles of Behaviour*. New York: Appleton-Century-Crofts.

Hunt, S.M. and Martin, C.J. (1988) Health-related behavioural change – a test of a new model. *Psychology and Health*, 2:209–30.

Illich, I. (1976) *Limits to Medicine*. Harmondsworth: Penguin.

Ingham, R. (1993) Old bodies in older clothes. *Health Psychology Update*, 14:31–6.

Janis, I.I. (1982) *Groupthink: Psychological Studies of Policy Decisions and Fiascoes*, 2nd edn. Boston, MA: Houghton Mifflin.

Johnston, M. (1982) Recognition of patients' worries by nurses and by other patients. *British Journal of Clinical Psychology*, 21:255–61.

Kanner, A.D., Coyne, J.C., Schaefer, C. and Lazarus, R.S. (1981) Comparison of two modes of stress measurement: Daily hassles and uplifts versus major life events. *Journal of Behavioral Medicine*, 4:1–39.

Kelly, G. (1955) *A Theory of Personality – The Psychology of Personal Constructs*. New York: Norton.

Kennel, J.H., Voos, D.K. and Klaus, M.H. (1979) Parent–infant bonding, in J.D. Osofsky (ed.), *Handbook of Infant Development*. New York: John Wiley.

Kleinhesselink, R.R. and Edwards, R.E. (1975) Seeking and avoiding belief-discrepant information as a function of its perceived refutability. *Journal of Personality and Social Psychology*, 31:787–90.

Kleinman, A. (1980) *Patients and Healers in the Context of Culture*. Berkeley, CA: University of California Press.

Kobasa, S.C. (1979) Stressful life events, personality and hardiness: An inquiry into hardiness. *Journal of Personality and Social Psychology*, 37:1–11.

Kogan, N. and Wallach, M.A. (1967) The risky-shift phenomenon in small decision-making groups: A test of the information exchange hypothesis. *Journal of Experimental Social Psychology*, 3:75–85.

Koster, M.E.T.A. and Bergsma, J. (1990) Problems and coping behaviour of facial cancer patients. *Social Science and Medicine*, 30(5):569–78.

Kubler-Ross, E. (1969) *On Death and Dying*. London: Tavistock.

Langer, E.J., and Rodin, J. (1976) The effects of choice and enhanced personal responsibility for the aged: A field experiment in an institutional setting. *Journal of Personality and Social Psychology*, 34(2):191–8.

Latané, B. and Darley, J.M. (1968) Group inhibition of bystander intervention in emergencies. *Journal of Personality and Social Psychology*, 10:215–21.

Latané, B. and Darley, J.M. (1970) *The Unresponsive Bystander: Why Does He not Help?* New York: Appleton-Century-Crofts.

Lau, R.R. and Hartman, K.A. (1983) Common sense representations of common illness. *Health Psychology*, 2:319–32.

Lawler, J. (1991) *Behind the Screens: Somology and the Problem of the Body*. London: Churchill Livingstone.

Lazarus, R.S. (1966) *Psychological Stress and the Coping Process*. New York: McGraw-Hill.

Lazarus, R.S. and Folkman, S. (1984) *Stress, Appraisal and Coping*. New York: Springer-Verlag.

Levenson, H. (1974) Activism and powerful others: Distinctions within the concept of internal–external control. *Journal of Personality Assessment*, 38:377–83.

Leventhal, H. and Nerenz, D. (1982) Representations of threat and the control of stress, in D. Meichenbaum and J. Jaremko (eds), *Stress Management and Prevention: A Cognitive-Behavioral Approach*. New York: Plenum Press.

Lewinsohn, P.M. (1974) Clinical and theoretical aspects of depression, in K.S. Calhoun, H.E. Adams and K.M. Mitchell (eds), *Innovative Methods in Psychopathology*. New York: John Wiley.

Ley, P. (1988) *Communicating with Patients: Improving Satisfaction and Compliance*. London: Chapman and Hall.

Linton, S.J. (1985) The relationship between activity and chronic back pain. *Pain*, 21:289–94.

Linville, P.W. (1987) Self-complexity as a cognitive buffer against stress-related illness and depression. *Journal of Personality and Social Psychology*, 52:663–76.

Littlewood, J. (1992) *Aspects of Grief*. London: Routledge.

MacGregor, F.C. (1970) Social and psychological implications of dentofacial disfigurement. *Angle Orthodontist*, 40:231–3.

Main, M. and Soloman, J. (1986) Discovery of an insecure disorganized attachment pattern, in T. Brazelton and M. Yogman (eds), *Affective Development in Infancy*. Norwood, NJ: Ablex.

Marks, D.F. (1994) *The Quit for Life Programme*. Leicester: British Psychological Society.

Maslow, A.H. (1970) *Motivation and Personality*, 2nd edn. New York: Harper and Row.

Mason, J.W. (1971) A re-evaluation of the concept of non-specificity in stress theory. *Journal of Psychiatric Research*, 8:323–33.

McCaffery, M. and Beebe, A. (eds) (1994) *Pain: Clinical Manual for Nursing Practice*. London: C.V. Mosby.

McLean, J. and Pietroni, P. (1990) Self care – who does best? *Social Science and Medicine*, 30(5):591–6.

Melzack, R. and Wall, P.D. (1988) *The Challenge of Pain*, 2nd edn. Harmondsworth: Penguin.

Miaskowski, C. (1994) Pain management: Quality assurance and changing practice, in M.R. Bond, J.E. Charlton and C.J. Woolf (eds), *Proceedings of the 7th World Congress on Pain*. Seattle: IASP.

Miller, J.F. (1992) *Coping with Chronic Illness: Overcoming Powerlessness*, 2nd edn. Philadelphia, PA: F.A. Davis.

Mills, M.A. and Walker, J.M. (1994) Memory, mood and dementia: A case study. *Journal of Aging Studies*, 8(1):17–27.

Mirowsky, J. and Ross, C.E. (1989) *Social Causes of Psychological Distress*. New York: Aldine de Gruyter.

Moos, R.H. (1974) Evaluating treatment environments. *Archives of General Psychiatry*, 26:414–18.

Morris, T., Pettingale, K. and Haybittle, J. (1992) Psychological response to cancer diagnosis and disease outcome in patients with breast cancer and lymphoma. *Psycho-oncology*, 1:105–14.

Moskovici, S. and Zavalloni, M. (1969) The group as a polarizer of attitudes. *Journal of Personality and Social Psychology*, 12:125–35.

Murray, M. (1990) Lay representations of illness, in P. Bennett, J. Weinman and P. Spurgeon (eds), *Current Developments in Health Psychology*, pp. 63–92. London: Harwood Academic.

Nelson, K. (ed.) (1986) *Event Knowledge: Structure and Function in Development*. Hillsdale, NJ: Lawrence Erlbaum Associates.

Nicholas, P.K. (1993) Hardiness, self-care practices and perceived health status in older adults. *Journal of Advanced Nursing*, 18:1085–94.

Oakley, A. (1992) *Social Support and Motherhood*. Oxford: Blackwell.

Owen, H., Plummer, J.L., Hopkins, L. and Cushnie, J. (1991) A comparison of nurse-administered and patient-controlled analgesia, in M.R. Bond, J.E. Charlton and C.J. Woolf (eds), *Proceedings of the VIth World Congress on Pain*. Amsterdam: Elsevier.

Parkes, C.M. (1986) *Bereavement: Studies in Grief in Adult Life*, 2nd edn. Penguin: Harmondsworth.

Parry, G. (1990) *Coping with Crises*. Leicester: British Psychological Society/Routledge.

Parsons, T. (1951) *The Social System*. Glencoe, IL: Free Press.

Passman, R.H. and Halonen, J.S. (1979) A developmental survey of young children's attachment to inanimate objects. *Journal of Genetic Psychology*, 134:165–78.

Payne, S. (1990) Lay representations of breast cancer. *Psychology and Health*, 5:1–11.

Payne, S. and Relf, M. (1994) The assessment of need for bereavement follow-up in palliative and hospice care. *Palliative Medicine*, 8(4):291–7.

Pennington, D.C. (1986) *Essential Social Psychology*. London: Edward Arnold.

Peterson, C. and Stunkard, A.J. (1989) Personal control and health promotion. *Social Science and Medicine*, 28(8):819–28.

Price, B. (1990) *Body Image: Nursing Concepts and Care*. New York: Prentice-Hall.

Price, B. (1994) The special needs of children. *Journal of Advanced Nursing*, 20:227–32.

Radley, A. (1994) *Making Sense of Illness*. London: Sage.

Raps, C.S., Jonas, M., Peterson, C. and Seligman, M.E.P. (1982) Patient behaviour in hospitals: Helplessness, reactance, or both? *Journal of Personality and Social Psychology*, 42(6):1036–41.

Reason, J. (1987) The Chernobyl errors. *Bulletin of the British Psychological Society*, 40:201–6.

Rosenberg, M. (1965) *Society and the Adolescent Self Image*. Princeton, NJ: Princeton University Press.

Rosenstiel, A.K. and Keefe, F.J. (1983) The use of coping strategies in chronic low back pain patients: Relationship to patient characteristics and current adjustment. *Pain*, 17:33–44.

Rosenstock, I.M. (1974a) Historical origins of the health belief model. *Health Education Monographs*, 2:328–35.

Rosenstock, I.M. (1974b) The health belief model and preventive health behaviour. *Health Education Monographs*, 2:354–86.

Rosenthal, R. (1966) *Experimenter Effects in Behavioural Research*. New York: Appleton-Century-Crofts.

Rosenthal, R. and Jacobson, L. (1968) *Pygmalion in the Classroom*. New York: Holt, Rinehart and Winston.

Ross, C.E. and Mirowsky, J. (1989) Explaining the social patterns of depression: Control and problem solving – or support and talking? *Journal of Health and Social Behaviour*, 30(2):206–19.

Rotter, J.B. (1966) Generalised expectancies for internal versus external control of reinforcement. *Psychological Monographs*, 80:1–28.

Roy, R. (1992) *The Social Context of the Chronic Pain Sufferer*. Toronto: University of Toronto Press.

Rutter, M. (1981) *Maternal Deprivation Reassessed*, 2nd edn. Harmondsworth: Penguin.

Sarason, B.R., Sarason, I.G. and Pierce, G.R. (eds) (1990) *Social Support: An Interactional View*. Chichester: John Wiley.

Schaffer, D.R. (1988) *Social and Personality Development*, 2nd edn. Pacific Grove, CA: Brooks/Cole.

Schaffer, H.R. and Emerson, P.E. (1964) Patterns of response to early physical contact in early human development. *Journal of Child Psychology and Psychiatry*, 5:1–13.

Schulz, K.H. and Schulz, H. (1992) Overview of psychoneuroimmunological stress and intervention studies in humans with emphasis on the uses of immunological parameters. *Psycho-oncology*, 1:51–70.

Seers, C. (1989) Patients' perceptions of acute pain, in J. Wilson-Barnett and S. Robinson (eds), *Directions in Nursing Research: Ten Years of Progress at London University*. London: Scutari.

Seers, K. and Davis, P. (1993) Pain in the nursing curriculum, in D. Carrol and D. Bowsher (eds), *Pain: Management and Nursing Care*. Oxford: Butterworth Heinemann.

Seligman, M.E.P. (1971) Phobias and preparedness. *Behaviour Therapy*, 2:307–20.

Seligman, M.E.P. (1975) *Helplessness: On Development, Depression and Death*. New York: Freeman.

Selye, H. (1956) *The Stress of Life*. New York: McGraw-Hill.

Schapiro, D.A. and Shapiro, D. (1982) Meta-analysis of comparative therapy outcome studies: A replication and refinement. *Psychological Bulletin*, 92:581–604.

Silverman, D., Bor, R., Miller, R. and Goldman, E. (1992) AIDS counselling: The interactional organization of talk about 'delicate' issues, in P. Aggleton, P. Davies and G. Hart (eds), *AIDS: Rights, Risks and Reason*. London: Falmer Press.

Simmons, S. (1994) Social networks: Their relevance to mental health nursing. *Journal of Advanced Nursing*, 19:281–9.

Skevington, S.M. (1983) Chronic pain and depression: Universal or personal helplessness? *Pain*, 15:309–17.

Slade, P., Williams, E. and Bartzokas, C. (1990) Changing health professional behaviour to reduce hospital-acquired infection. Paper presented at the *British Psychological Society Conference*, London, December.

Snelling, J. (1994) The effect of chronic pain on the family unit. *Journal of Advanced Nursing*, 19:543–51.

Sofaer, B. (1985) Pain management through nurse education, in L.A. Copp (ed.), *Perspectives on Pain*. Edinburgh: Churchill Livingstone.

Spieker, S.J. and Bensley, L. (1994) Roles of living arrangements and grandmother social support in adolescent mothering and infant attachment. *Developmental Psychology*, 30(1):102–11.

Sque, M. and Payne, S.A. (1994) The experiences of donor families. Paper presented at the *Palliative Care Research Forum*, Dublin, November.

Stainton Rogers, W. (1991) *Explaining Health and Illness: An Exploration of Diversity*. Hemel Hempstead: Harvester Wheatsheaf.

Sternbach, R.A. and Timmermans, G. (1975) Personality changes associated with reduction of pain. *Pain*, 1:177–81.

Stetz, K.M., Lewis, F.M. and Primomo, J. (1986) Family coping strategies and chronic illness in the mother. *Family Relations*, 35:515–22.

Stroebe, M.S. (1994) *Helping the Bereaved Come to Terms with Loss: What Does Bereavement Research Have to Offer?* St George's Mental Health Library Conference Series. London: St George's Hospital.

Taylor, S.E. (1991) *Health Psychology*, 2nd edn. New York: McGraw-Hill.

Teasdale, K. (ed.) (1992) *Managing the Changes in Health Care*. London: Wolfe.

Temoshok, L. (1987) Personality, coping style, emotion and cancer: Towards an integrative model. *Cancer Surveys*, 6(iii):545–67.

Thorne, B. (1992) *Carl Rogers*. London: Sage.

Vachon, M.L.S., Rogers, J., Lyall, W.A.L., Lancee, W.J., Sheldon, A.R. and Freeman, S.J.J. (1982) Predictors and correlates of adaptation to conjugal bereavement. *American Journal of Psychiatry*, 139:998–1002.

Waddell, G. (1992) Biopsychosocial analysis of low back pain. *Bailliere's Clinical Rheumatology*, 6(3):523–51.

Walker, J.M. (1989) The management of elderly patients with pain: A community nursing perspective. Unpublished PhD Thesis, Bournemouth University.

Walker, J.M. (1993) A social behavioural approach to understanding and promoting condom use, in J. Wilson-Barnett and J. Macleod Clark (eds), *Research in Health Promotion and Nursing*. Basingstoke: Macmillan.

Walker, J.M., Akinsanya, J.A., Davis, B.D. and Marcer, D.M. (1990) The nursing management of elderly patients with pain in the community: Study and recommendations. *Journal of Advanced Nursing*, 15:1154–61.

Wallston, K.A., Wallston, B.S. and DeVellis, R. (1978) Development of the Multidimensional Health Locus of Control (MHLOC) scale. *Health Education Monographs*, 6(2):161–70.

Webb, C. (1989) Action research: Philosophy, methods and personal experiences. *Journal of Advanced Nursing*, 14:403–10.

Westmacott, E.V.S. and Cameron, R.J. (1981) *Behaviour Can Change*. London: Macmillan.

Williams, A.C. de C., Ralphs, J.A., Nicholas, M.K., Richardson, P.H. *et al.* (1993) A cognitive behavioural programme for rehabilitating the chronic pain patient: Result of the first 200 cases. *British Journal of General Practice*, 43:513–18.

Wolf, Z.R. (1986) Nurses' work: The sacred and the profane. *Holistic Nursing Practice*, 1(1):29–35.

Wolpe, J. (1958) *Psychotherapy by Reciprocal Inhibition*. Stanford, CA: Stanford University Press.

Wortman, C.B. and Silver, R.C. (1989) The myths of coping with loss. *Journal of Consulting and Clinical Psychology*, 57(3):349–57.

Zola, I. (1972) Medicine as an institution of social control. *Sociological Review*, 20:487–504.

INDEX